KETO AIR FRYER COOKBOOK

Low-carb Air Fryer Recipes That Will Make Eating Healthy

(Quick and Easy Ketogenic Diet Friendly Air Fryer Recipes)

Patricia Parks

I0092613

Published by Sharon Lohan

© **Patricia Parks**

All Rights Reserved

Keto Air Fryer Cookbook: Low-carb Air Fryer Recipes That Will Make Eating Healthy (Quick and Easy Ketogenic Diet Friendly Air Fryer Recipes)

ISBN 978-1-990334-01-6

All rights reserved. No part of this guide may be reproduced in any form without permission in writing from the publisher except in the case of brief quotations embodied in critical articles or reviews.

Legal & Disclaimer

The information contained in this book is not designed to replace or take the place of any form of medicine or professional medical advice. The information in this book has been provided for educational and entertainment purposes only.

The information contained in this book has been compiled from sources deemed reliable, and it is accurate to the best of the Author's knowledge; however, the Author cannot guarantee its accuracy and validity and cannot be held liable for any errors or omissions. Changes are periodically made to this book. You must consult your doctor or get professional medical advice before using any of the suggested remedies, techniques, or information in this book.

Table of contents

Part 1

Introduction

Throughout the better part of the past 100 years, the ketogenic diet has been a quintessential answer to weight loss. Unlike other diets, the ketogenic diet isn't about "counting calories" or even exercising. Rather, it involves counting the amount of carbohydrates you take in to make sure that your body resorts to using its stored fat for energy, rather than the sugars you might have otherwise eaten on any other "normal-carbohydrate diet."

Each of the following 50 recipes restricts your normal carbohydrate intake, upping your protein and fat intake to create "ketosis" in your body. This means that the amount of glucose in your body (what's found in carb-heavy foods, like sugar, fruit, grains, and breads) is restricted. Each recipe in this book has no more than 15 grams of carbohydrates per serving, meaning that you can restrict your carb levels to under 50 grams each day—a recommended amount to remain in ketosis.

In fact, when first starting out on ketosis, it's recommended to begin in the 30 to 50 grams of carbohydrates range.

Plus, each recipe includes the carb count AND the fiber count. The amount of carbs your body actually has to handle—the "net carbs"—are the carb count minus the fiber count. Not to mention, each recipe also includes the fat, protein and calorie counts, meaning you CAN keep track of those things, if you want to, on your weight loss journey.

And the air fryer is one of the most beneficial tools in the kitchen: helping you to make low-calorie and nutritionally rich recipes, all without taking too much time out of your day.

Good luck on your journey, and trust the process. The minute your body enters ketosis, you'll start seeing results. It's science.

Ketogenic Air Fryer Breakfast Recipes

No Egg Vegan Air Fryer Breakfast Scramble

Recipe Makes 4 Servings.
Preparation Time: 25 minutes

Nutritional Information Per Serving: 206 calories, 15 grams carbohydrates, 13 grams fat, 12 grams protein, 4 grams fiber.

Ingredients:
1 diced onion
1 chopped carrot
1 tsp. olive oil
1/2 cup diced green pepper
2 chopped celery stalks
1 tsp. dried oregano
3/4 cup diced shiitake mushrooms
1/2 tsp. salt
1/2 tsp. pepper
1/2 tsp. red pepper flakes
1/2 tsp. dried dill
8 oz. tofu, drained and extra firm
2 tbsp. soy yogurt
2 tbsp. nutritional yeast
1 tbsp. lemon juice
2 tbsp. water

Directions:

First, pour the olive oil into a skillet and heat over medium-high. Then, add the garlic, and the onion, and cook for about five minutes, or until the onion is see-through.

Next, add the celery, carrot, and the bell pepper, and sauté the mixture for another four minutes. Add the spices and the mushrooms at this time, and cook for another three minutes, stirring well.

To the side, pulse together the nutritional yeast, soy yogurt, water, lemon juice, and the tofu. The mixture should be creamy.

Pour the tofu mixture into the skillet. Stir well.

Next, pour the mixture into a baking dish (that fits in the air fryer), and bake the scramble at 350 degrees Fahrenheit for 15 minutes.

The mixture should be golden brown. Serve the vegan scramble warm, and enjoy.

Cheddar and Sausage Breakfast Frittata

Recipe Makes 1 Serving.
Preparation Time: 20 minutes

Nutritional Information Per Serving: 460 calories, 4.5 grams carbohydrates, 41 grams fat, 22 grams protein, 1 gram fiber.

Ingredients:
2 eggs
1 tbsp. chopped onions
2 tbsp. shredded cheddar cheese
1 chopped patty of sausage
1 tbsp. butter, melted
2 tbsp. chopped green peppers
1/2 tsp. salt
1/2 tsp. pepper

Butter or olive oil to grease a cake pan for cooking

Directions:
Preheat the air fryer to 350 degrees Fahrenheit for five minutes.

Next, use some butter or olive oil to smear on the bottom of a four-inch cake pan or a small loaf pan.

Next, chop up your piece of sausage and place it at the bottom of the small pan, making it even across the pan. Cook the sausage in the air fryer for five minutes.

Next, to the side in a medium-sized bowl, crack the eggs and whisk them with a fork. Add pepper and salt and whisk until well combined.

Add the green peppers and the onions to the eggs and stir well. Then, pour the egg mixture over the top of the sausage, and stir well.

Sprinkle the cheddar cheese over the top of the eggs, and then air fry the frittata for a full five minutes in the preheated air fryer.

Serve the frittata warm, and enjoy.

Mother's Best Bacon Cups with Eggs

Recipe Makes 4 Servings.
Preparation Time: 15 minutes

Nutritional Information Per Serving: 270 calories, 1 gram carbohydrate, 19 grams protein, 20 grams fat, 0 grams fiber.

Ingredients:
8 bacon rashers

1 tsp. salt

1 tsp. pepper

4 eggs

4 ramekins for cooking the eggs and bacon together

Directions:

Preheat the air fryer to 400 degrees Fahrenheit.

First, add the bacon around the sides and the bottoms of each of the ramekins, so that it creates a kind of "crust" or "cone."

Then, crack each egg into the center of each ramekin, and place the ramekins in the air fryer.

Cook them in the air fryer for 13 minutes. Then, season with salt and pepper, and serve warm.

Air Fried Radish "Hashbrowns"

Recipe Makes 4 Servings.
Preparation Time: 24 minutes

Nutritional Information Per Serving: 64 calories, 7 grams carbohydrates, 1 gram protein, 4 grams fat, 3 grams fiber.

Ingredients:
1 pound radishes
1 tsp. garlic powder
1 diced onion
1 tsp. sea salt
1 tsp. onion powder
1/2 tsp. black pepper
1/2 tsp. paprika
1 tbsp. coconut oil

Directions:
First, wash the radishes and then slice off the ends of them, at the root. Then, use a food processor to slice both the radishes and the onions.

Melt the coconut oil at this time, either in the microwave or on the stove, and pour the coconut oil in with the onions and the radishes, and stir well.

At this time, grease the interior of the air fryer basket, and add the onions and the radishes to the interior.

Then, cook the radishes and the onions in the air fryer for eight minutes at 350 degrees Fahrenheit. Make sure to shake it every few minutes as it cooks, to move the vegetables around.

Next, pour the radish and onion mixture back into the bowl, and stir well. Add the sea salt, onion powder, garlic powder, black pepper, and paprika, and then stir well to assimilate the spices.

Serve the radishes and onion hash browns warm, and enjoy.

Crispy Keto Bacon

Recipe Makes 8 pieces of bacon
Preparation Time: 6 minutes

Nutritional Information Per Serving (2 strips of bacon each): 205 calories, .5 grams carbohydrates, 14 grams protein, 15 grams fat, 0 grams fiber.

Ingredients:
8 strips of bacon

Directions:

First, place four strips of bacon at the bottom of the air fryer. Place the wire rack over the top of the bacon, and cook the bacon at 390 degrees Fahrenheit for three minutes.

Then, open up the air fryer and flip the bacon. Cook for an additional three minutes. Remove the strips of bacon and repeat these steps with the rest of the bacon.

Do so until you've had your fill of bacon. Serve warm and crispy, and enjoy.

Ketogenic Air Fryer Chicken Recipes

Southern Fried Chicken

Recipe Makes 8 Servings.
Preparation Time: 60 minutes to marinate, plus 8 minutes

Nutritional Information Per Serving: 256 calories, 1.3 grams carbohydrates, 34 grams protein, 11.6 grams fat, .4 grams fiber.

Ingredients:
2 pounds of chicken thighs
2 tsp. garlic powder
1/2 tsp. chili powder
1/2 tsp. paprika
1 egg
1/2 cup almond flour
2 tbsp. heavy cream
1/3 cup grated Parmesan

Directions:
Slice the chicken into smaller, easy to handle and eat pieces, and add them to a mixing bowl.

Next, coat the chicken with the garlic powder, chili powder, and the paprika, and let the chicken marinate in the spices for over an hour.

Preheat the air fryer to 400 degrees Fahrenheit at this time. Afterwards, stir together the cream and the eggs in a medium-sized bowl.

To the side, stir together the Parmesan and the almond flour in a medium-sized bowl.

Now, prep your chicken by dipping the chicken pieces into the egg, then rolling them in the almond and Parmesan cheese. Set each piece to the side until you've prepped every piece.

Next, add the chicken to the basket. Fry the chicken in the air fryer for eight minutes, or until each piece is golden brown. If you're not sure if they're done, simply remove a piece of chicken and slice it at its thickest point to make sure.

Serve the fried chicken warm, and enjoy.

Chicken and Vegetable Kebabs

Recipe Makes 2 Servings.
Preparation Time: 25 minutes

Nutritional Information Per Serving: 315 calories, 20 grams carbohydrates, 33.5 grams protein, 11 grams fat, 3.2 grams fiber.

Ingredients:
1/3 cup agave nectar
1/3 cup soy sauce
6 sliced mushrooms
3 sliced green and red peppers
1 tsp. salt
1 tsp. pepper

2 diced chicken breasts
1 tbsp. olive oil

Wooden skewers for making the kebabs

Directions:
First, dice the chicken breasts and dot them with salt and pepper. Next, stir together the agave nectar, olive oil, and the soy sauce in a small bowl.

Next, place the chicken, peppers, and mushrooms on wooden skewers, making sure to alternate.

Preheat the air fryer to 340 degrees Fahrenheit for five minutes. During this time, coat the skewer chicken kebabs with the sauce.

Then, place the kebabs in the air fryer basket. Cook them for 20 minutes.

Then, allow the chicken kebabs to cool for a few minutes before serving.

Chicken Tenders Made with Buttermilk

Recipe Makes 4 Servings.
Preparation Time: 23 minutes

Nutritional Information Per Serving: 253 calories, 7 grams carbohydrates, 13 grams fat, 24 grams protein, 2.2 grams fiber.

Ingredients:
8 oz. chicken breasts, boneless and skinless
1 cup buttermilk
2 cups almond flour
2 eggs
1 tbsp. paprika
1 tbsp. sea salt
1/2 tbsp. parsley

Directions:
First, place the chicken breasts between two pieces of kitchen plastic wrap. Then, use a rolling pin to bang out the chicken until they're about a half an inch thick. Then, slice the chicken into strips of approximately one inch across.

Place the chicken strips inside of a bowl and pour the buttermilk over them, making sure to cover them. Allow them to marinate in the buttermilk for a full hour.

Next, stir together the almond flour, parsley, paprika, and the salt in another large bowl. In a separate bowl, beat together the eggs.

Next, dredge each of the chicken strips in the egg, and then dredge them in the salt mixture. Add each chicken strip to the air fryer basket. When you've added each one, cook the chicken at 350 degrees Fahrenheit for three minutes.

Afterwards, shake the basket well, making sure that the chicken flips. Then, cook for an additional four minutes.

Afterwards, the chicken should be a golden brown color, and crispy. Make sure that the internal temperature of the chicken is 165 degrees Fahrenheit. Find out by inserting a meat thermometer into the center.

Remove the chicken from the basket and serve warm.

Chicken Parmesan

Recipe Makes 4 Servings.
Preparation Time: 30 minutes

Nutritional Information Per Serving: 316 calories, 5.3 grams carbohydrates, 36 grams protein, 15.1 grams fat, 1 gram fiber.

Ingredients:
2 chicken breasts, sliced in half
3 tbsp. almond flour
3 tbsp. Parmesan cheese, grated
3 tbsp. mozzarella cheese, shredded
1 tbsp. olive oil
1/2 cup marinara sauce

Directions:
First, preheat the air fryer to 360 degrees Fahrenheit, making sure it heats for nine minutes.

Next, stir together the almond flour and the Parmesan cheese in a large bowl.

To the side, add the olive oil in another bowl. Glaze the chicken with the olive oil, and then dip the chicken in the almond flour and Parmesan, coating it completely.

Afterwards, place two pieces of the chicken in the air fryer basket and cook for six minutes. Then, turn the chicken and top them each with one tbsp. of marinara sauce, followed by about 2 tbsp. of mozzarella cheese. Allow the chicken to cook for three more minutes.

Now, remove them from the air fryer, and repeat these steps with the two additional chicken pieces.

Serve the chicken warm, and enjoy.

Tandoori Chicken

Recipe Makes 4 Servings.
Preparation Time: 45 minutes

Nutritional Information Per Serving: 325 calories, 3.5 grams carbohydrates, 43 grams protein, 14.4 grams fat, .7 grams fiber.

Ingredients:
1 1/4 pound chicken tenders, sliced into halves
1 tbsp. minced garlic
1/3 cup Greek yogurt, unflavored and plain
1 tsp. sea salt
1 tbsp. minced ginger
1 tsp. cayenne pepper
1 tsp. paprika, smoked
1/2 tsp. garam masala
1 1/2 tsp. turmeric

1 tbsp. lemon juice
1 tbsp. ghee
2 tbsp. chopped cilantro

Directions:

First, stir together the minced garlic, Greek yogurt, sea salt, minced ginger, cayenne pepper, paprika, garam masala, and turmeric in a medium-sized bowl. Place the pieces of sliced chicken into the mixture and coat it well, stirring it into the mixture.

Allow the chicken to sit for 25 minutes in the marinade. After 25 minutes, preheat the air fryer to 350 degrees Fahrenheit for five minutes.

After five minutes, open the air fryer, and place the chicken pieces in one layer on the rack of your air fryer.

Next, use a brush to brush the ghee on top of the chicken on a single side. Cook the chicken for ten minutes in the preheated air fryer.

Then, remove the chicken and flip them over, brushing the other side with the ghee.
Cook the chicken for an additional five minutes.

Afterwards, use a meat thermometer to ensure that the chicken has reached a temperature of 165 degrees Fahrenheit on the inside.

Next, remove the chicken and place it on a platter. Top the chicken with the lemon juice and the cilantro, and serve warm.

An Entire Rotisserie Chicken

Recipe Makes 4 Servings.
Preparation Time: 1 hour and 10 minutes

Nutritional Information Per Serving: 224 calories, 4.4 grams carbohydrates, 35 grams protein, 7.8 grams fat, 0.3 grams fiber.

Ingredients:
1 chicken, washed and patted dry
1 tsp. garlic powder
1 tsp. onion powder
1 tsp. dried parsley
1 tsp. sea salt
1 tsp. black pepper
2 tbsp. coconut oil

Directions:
First, remove the giblet from the chicken and pat the chicken dry.

Next, rub the coconut oil over the chicken, making sure to coat it. Then, season the chicken with the onion powder, garlic powder, dried parsley, black pepper,

20

and the sea salt. Make sure to rub the spices all over the chicken.

Then, place the chicken inside the air fryer with the breast down.

Next, cook the chicken at 350 degrees Fahrenheit. Do so for 30 minutes.

Afterwards, flip the chicken so that the breast is up, and cook at the same temperature for another 30 minutes. The inside of the chicken should reach a temperature of 165 degrees. Make sure to use your meat thermometer to check.

Allow the chicken to rest after cooking for ten minutes, and then serve warm.

Chicken Roll-Ups with Veggies

Recipe Makes 4 Servings.
Preparation Time: 20 minutes

Nutritional Information Per Serving: 245 calories, 3.7 grams carbohydrates, 44.5 grams protein, 4.9 grams fat, 1 gram fiber.

Ingredients:
3 chicken breasts

2 tsp. paprika

1/2 sliced green pepper

1/2 sliced yellow pepper

1/2 sliced red pepper

1 tsp. garlic powder

1/2 tsp. cayenne pepper

1 tsp. onion powder

1 tsp. cumin powder

1/2 tsp. oregano

1/2 tsp. salt

1/2 tsp. Pepper

Toothpicks, for rolling up the chicken

Directions:

First, stir together the spices: the paprika, garlic powder, cayenne pepper, onion powder, cumin powder, oregano, and the salt and pepper in a small bowl. Put the bowl to the side at this time.

Next, slice the chicken breasts into two pieces.

Next, place each half of chicken breast between two pieces of parchment paper. Then, use a rolling pin to smash at the chicken to flatten it out. You should bang at it until its thickness is a quarter of an inch.

Next, season the chicken with the spice mixture from above. Do this liberally, rubbing it into the skin of the chicken.

Then, place the bell pepper pieces on one side of each piece of chicken. Then, roll up the chicken like a "roll up," and secure the chicken roll ups with toothpicks.

Then, repeat this process with each of the pieces of chicken. Sprinkle whatever you have left of the spice mixture over the chicken.

Then, place the chicken in the air fryer basket, and air fry the chicken at 400 degrees Fahrenheit for 12 minutes. Serve the chicken roll-ups warm, and enjoy.

Asian Chicken Wings

Recipe Makes 4 Servings.
Preparation Time: 25 minutes

Nutritional Information Per Serving: 487 calories, 3.7 grams carbohydrates, 21.5 grams fat, 66 grams protein, .2 grams fiber.

Ingredients:
2 pounds of chicken wings, with the bones
1 tsp. pepper
1 tsp. salt

Sauce ingredients:
1 tbsp. sesame oil
1 tbsp. mayonnaise
2 tbsp. minced garlic
1 tsp. maple syrup

Directions:
First, preheat the air fryer to 400 degrees Fahrenheit for ten minutes.

Next, line a small baking pan with aluminum foil, and place the air fryer rack within the baking pan.

Next, pepper and salt the chicken wings well, and place them on the air fryer rack.

Cook the chicken wings for twenty minutes in the air fryer, turning once at the halfway point.

As you air fry the chicken, stir together the sesame oil, mayonnaise, minced garlic, and the maple syrup in a medium-sized bowl. Allow the sauce to sit while the chicken cooks.

After the chicken timer's up, make sure the interior of the chicken is 160 degrees Fahrenheit by using a thermometer.

If it's reached this temperature, toss the wings with half of the sauce. Then, cook the chicken wings for an additional five minutes.

Serve the chicken with the rest of the sauce over the top, and enjoy.

Keto Friendly Chicken Cordon Bleu

Recipe Makes 2 Servings.
Preparation Time: 14 minutes

Nutritional Information Per Serving: 494 calories, 5.1 grams carbohydrates, 74 grams protein, 18 grams fat, 1.8 grams fiber.

Ingredients:
2 medium-sized chicken breasts
1 slice of cheddar cheese

1 slice of ham

1 tbsp. of cream cheese, or another soft cheese

1/2 cup almond flour

1 tbsp. thyme, fresh and chopped

1 tbsp. tarragon,

1 tsp. dried parsley

1 tsp. garlic powder

1/2 tsp. salt

1/2 tsp. pepper

Directions:

First, preheat the air fryer to 400 degrees Fahrenheit.

Next, place the chicken breasts on a cutting board, and slide your knife through the center of them, at an angle, so that you can open them up and stuff them.

Next, sprinkle the pepper, tarragon, and salt on the inside of the chicken.

To the side, stir together the parsley, soft cheese, and garlic powder together in a small bowl. When it's well-mixed, add a layer of this mixture to the inside of the chicken. Then, top this layer of soft cheese with half a slice of cheddar cheese, and a half a slice of the ham (with one half for each of the chicken breasts).

Next, press down on the top of the chicken to seal it.

To the side, add the egg to a small bowl, and add the almond flour to another bowl. Stir the egg with a fork to make it "scrambled."

Then, roll the chicken in the egg, and then in the almond flour to coat it well.

Next, place the chicken on a baking sheet in the air fryer. Cook the chicken for 30 minutes. At the 20 minute marker, turn over the chicken to ensure that the chicken is crispy on all sides.

Serve warm, and enjoy.

Air Fryer Turkey Breast with Rosemary

Recipe Makes 6 Servings.
Preparation Time: 35 minutes

Nutritional Information Per Serving: 469 calories, 8.9 grams carbohydrates, 55 grams protein, 22 grams fat, 1 gram fiber.

Ingredients:
2 1/2 pounds turkey
2 tsp. chopped rosemary
3 minced garlic cloves
1/3 cup olive oil

3 tbsp. agave nectar
2 tsp. sea salt
1 tbsp. brown mustard
1 tbsp. butter
1 tsp. crushed red pepper

Directions:

First, stir together the olive oil, rosemary, salt, and garlic in a small bowl.

Spread this mixture over the turkey, on both sides of the turkey breast. Cover the turkey and allow it to marinate for two hours—or even overnight, if you have the time.

Remove the turkey from the refrigerator about 30 minutes to an hour prior to cooking it.

Grease your air fryer basket with olive oil or butter, and add the turkey to the air fryer at this time. Cook it at 400 degrees Fahrenheit for a full 20 minutes.

Next, place one tbsp. of butter in a small bowl, and melt it for 10 seconds in a microwave. Add the agave nectar and the mustard to the butter and stir it well.

After the turkey's done with its first 20 minutes of cooking, add the mustard mixture over the top of the turkey, spreading it across the top to create a glaze.

Next, add the turkey back to the air fryer and cook for an additional 10 minutes at 400 degrees Fahrenheit.

Afterwards, remove the turkey from the air fryer and allow it to sit for 10 minutes. Then, slice the turkey against the grain and serve warm.

Turkey-Crust Pizza

Recipe Makes 6 Servings.
Preparation Time: 35 minutes

Nutritional Information Per Serving: 283 calories, 1.9 grams carbohydrates, 34 grams protein, 16.6 grams fat, 0.3 grams fiber.

Crust Ingredients:
1 1/4 pound ground turkey
1 egg
2 1/4 cup grated mozzarella cheese
1 tsp. garlic powder
1/2 tsp. onion powder

Topping Ingredients:
4 slices turkey bacon
2 tbsp. marinara sauce
6 black olives, sliced into pieces

1/2 cup mozzarella cheese, for topping
Any additional toppings you desire

Directions:
First, preheat the air fryer to 400 degrees Fahrenheit.

Next, stir together the crust ingredients: garlic powder, onion powder, ground turkey, and the mozzarella, and stir with your hands so that you don't "overwork" the turkey.

Next, press the mixture into a flat form, like a curst, and place the crust at the bottom of the air fryer. Air fry the crust for 15 minutes.

Next, remove the crust from heat, and add the tomato sauce, half of the mozzarella cheese, olives, and bacon. Add the rest of the cheese over the top, and then place the pizza back in the air fryer. Allow it to air fry for an additional 12 minutes.

At this time, allow the pizza to cool for about five minutes before enjoying.

Ketogenic Air Fryer Beef Recipes

Yummy Beef Meatballs

Recipe Makes 4 Servings.
Preparation Time: 15 minutes

Nutritional Information Per Serving: 279 calories, 3.5 grams carbohydrates, 12 grams fat, 37 grams protein, 1 gram fiber.

Ingredients:
1 pound ground beef
1/2 cup almond flour
2 tsp. onion powder
2 minced garlic cloves
2 tsp. garlic powder
1 egg
1/2 tsp. salt
1/2 tsp. pepper
2 tsp. olive oil

Directions:
First, in a medium-sized bowl, stir together the almond flour, onion powder, and the garlic powder. Add the salt and pepper and stir well.

Next, stir together the beef, garlic and the egg, using your hands so that you don't over-mix. Make the meatballs into golf ball-sized balls, and place them to the side, on a platter.

At this time, preheat your air fryer for five minutes at 400 degrees Fahrenheit.

Next, add a bit of olive oil to the bottom of the air fryer, and add the meatballs into the air fryer, making sure to leave space around each one so that they don't touch one another or the sides. You might need to do them in batches.

Next, cook the meatballs for ten minutes, and remove them and repeat the process with another batch. You can keep the meatballs warm in the oven as you cook the others.

Serve warm, and enjoy.

Air Fried Beef Burgers

Recipe Makes 4 Servings.
Preparation Time: 20 minutes

Nutritional Information Per Serving: 217 calories, 1.4 grams carbohydrates, 34 grams protein, 7.1 grams fat, 0 grams fiber.

Ingredients:
1 pound ground beef
1/2 tsp. onion powder
1/2 tsp. sea salt
1/2 tsp. dried oregano
1/2 tsp. garlic powder
1 tbsp. Worcestershire sauce
1 tsp. parsley, dried

Directions:
First, preheat the air fryer to 350 degrees Fahrenheit.

To the side, stir together the seasoning: the onion powder, dried oregano, garlic powder, sea salt, and parsley. Add the Worcestershire sauce, and stir well, before adding the beef.

Using your hands, work the meat to assimilate the various spices and herbs.

Next, divide the meat into four patties, and shape them, putting an indent in the very center of each burger patty to make sure the patties don't become too thick in the middle.

Next, place the burgers in the air fryer tray, and cook the burgers for ten minutes to get a medium doneness, longer if you prefer them well done. You don't need to turn the patties at any time.

Serve the burgers warm, and enjoy.

Air Fried Steak

Recipe Makes 2 Servings.
Preparation Time: 10 minutes

Nutritional Information Per Serving: 484 calories, 1 gram carbohydrate, 82 grams protein, 14 grams fat, 0.3 gram fiber.

Ingredients:
2 steaks, with a thickness of approximately one inch
1 tsp. sea salt
1 tsp. pepper
1/2 tbsp. olive oil

Directions:
First, place the baking tray in the air fryer and preheat the air fryer for five minutes at 450 degrees Fahrenheit.

Coat the steak with the olive oil, and then season both sides of the steak with both pepper and salt.

Next, place the steak in the air fryer baking tray, and cook for three minutes.

After three minutes, flip the steak to the other side and cook for an additional three minutes.

Remove the steak from the air fryer, and allow it to rest on a side plate for three minutes prior to serving. Serve warm, and enjoy.

Meatloaf

Recipe Makes 4 Servings.
Preparation Time: 25 minutes

Nutritional Information Per Serving: 293 calories, 3.8 grams carbohydrates, 42 grams protein, 11.5 grams fat, 1 gram fiber.

Ingredients:
1 pound of ground beef
1 cup pork rinds, crumbled
1 egg
1/2 diced onion
2 tsp. black pepper
2 tsp. salt
1 tsp. dried basil
2 minced garlic cloves
1/3 cup tomato sauce
1/2 cup grated Parmesan cheese

Directions:
First, preheat the air fryer to 350 degrees Fahrenheit.

Next, stir together the meat, egg, pork rinds, onion, black pepper, salt, dried basil, garlic cloves, tomato sauce, and the Parmesan cheese, using your hands to stir and assimilate so as not to overwork the meat.

When it's mixed well, form the meatloaf into a loaf-form.

Place the loaf in the air fryer basket, and air fry the meatloaf for 22 minutes. Afterwards, turn off the heat and carefully remove the meatloaf, allowing it to cool for a few minutes prior to serving.

Ketogenic Air Fryer Pork Recipes

Crunchy Pork Chops

Recipe Makes 6 Servings.
Preparation Time: 14 minutes

Nutritional Information Per Serving: 530 calories, 1 gram carbohydrate, 92 grams protein, 15 grams fat, 0.3 grams fiber.

Ingredients:
6 boneless pork chops, cut thick
1/2 tsp. black pepper
1/2 tsp. salt
1 tsp. paprika, smoked
2 eggs
1/2 tsp. chili powder
1/2 tsp. onion powder
1 cup of crumbs from crumbled-up pork rinds
4 tbsp. Parmesan cheese, grated

Directions:
First, preheat the air fryer to 400 degrees Fahrenheit. Allow it to heat for ten minutes prior to cooking.

Season the pork chops with pepper and salt. At this time, add the pork rinds to a food processor and blend them into crumbs.

Next, stir together the pork rinds, paprika, chili powder, onion powder, and the Parmesan cheese in a large mixing bowl.

Crack the eggs in a separate bowl. Dip the pork chops into the egg mixture, then dip them into the seasoning and Parmesan and pork rind mixture. Coat well.

Then, place the pork into the basket in the air fryer. When you've finished prepping each pork chop, cook them at 400 degrees Fahrenheit for about 15 minutes.

Afterwards, serve the pork chops warm, and enjoy.

Asian Pepper Pork Chops

Recipe Makes 4 Servings.
Preparation Time: 40 minutes

Nutritional Information Per Serving: 408 calories, 1 gram carbohydrate, 26 grams protein, 32 grams fat, 0 grams fiber.

Ingredients:

1 pound pork chops, sliced into smaller pieces
1 egg white
1/2 tsp. black pepper
1/2 tsp. sea salt
3/4 cup almond flour
1 tbsp. olive oil
Additional salt and pepper to taste

Directions:

First, add the olive oil to the bottom of the air fryer basket.

To the side, stir together the egg, pepper, and salt, using a fork to make it foamy.

Slice the pork chops into smaller pieces, and add them to the egg white mixture, coating the pork completely. Allow the pork to marinate for 20 minutes.

Next, place the pork chops in a large mixing bowl and add the almond flour, dredging them completely in the flour.

Shake off the pieces of pork, and place them in the air fryer basket. Cook the pork pieces for 12 minutes at a temperature of 355 degrees Fahrenheit, shaking the basket every minute or so.

After 12 minutes, increase the temperature to 400 degrees Fahrenheit, and cook for an additional six minutes to make the pork crispy. Shake well throughout the cooking process.

Serve the pork chops warm, and enjoy.

Mustard and Lemon Glazed Pork

Recipe Makes 4 Servings.
Preparation Time: 15 minutes

Nutritional Information Per Serving: 331 calories, 2.2 grams carbohydrates, 32 grams protein, 20 grams fat, 1 gram fiber.

Ingredients:
16 ounces pork loins
1 tsp. black pepper
1 tbsp. sea salt

1 tsp. thyme

1 tsp. paprika

Sauce Ingredients:

1 tsp. apple cider vinegar

1/3 cup heavy cream

1/2 cup chicken broth

1 tbsp. mustard

Juice from 1/2 lemon

Directions:

First, pat the pork loins dry using paper towels and then salt, pepper, thyme, and paprika them—making sure to coat both sides of the loins.

Next, place a skillet on high heat and brown the pork loins for about three minutes on both sides. Then, set the pork loins to the side.

Then, add the heavy cream, chicken broth and the apple cider vinegar to the skillet and allow it to simmer, deglazing the pot as it cooks with your spatula. Then, add the mustard and lemon juice, and stir well to combine.

Next, add the pork loins to the air fryer, and cover them with the mustard mixture. Allow them to cook in the air fryer for eight minutes at 400 degrees

Fahrenheit, making sure to flip them after four minutes.

Afterwards, serve the pork loins warm, with extra sauce glazed over the top.

Garlic Pork Chops

Recipe Makes 6 Servings.
Preparation Time: 20 minutes

Nutritional Information Per Serving: 536 calories, 2.6 grams carbohydrates, 28 grams protein, 45 grams fat, 0 grams fiber.

Ingredients:
1 1/2 pounds pork chops, without the bone
2 minced garlic cloves
1/2 diced onion
1 cup heavy cream
2 tbsp. olive oil
1/4 cup cream cheese
1/3 cup Parmesan cheese
1/3 cup chicken broth
1/2 tsp. black pepper

1/2 tsp. sea salt

1 tbsp. Italian seasoning

Directions:

First, add the garlic, olive oil, onion, and the pork chops to a large skillet and heat on high heat, browning the pork chops for five minutes on each side.

Then, remove the pork from the skillet, and add the rest of the ingredients to create a sauce. Stir as the sauce heats.

Just as the sauce begins to boil—after four minutes— remove the sauce from the heat, and place the pork in the air fryer. Pour the mixture over the pork, and air fry the pork for five minutes on 350 degrees Fahrenheit. Make sure to flip the pork halfway through cooking.

Serve the pork warm, with the sauce over the top.

Pork Chops with Parmesan Crust

Recipe Makes 6 Servings.
Preparation Time: 35 minutes

Nutritional Information Per Serving: 444 calories, .5 gram carbohydrates, 35 grams fat, 30 grams protein, 0 grams fiber.

Ingredients:
1 1/2 pounds pork chops
2 tbsp. olive oil
1/2 cup crushed pork rinds
1/2 cup Parmesan cheese, grated
1/2 tsp. minced garlic
1/2 tsp. lemon zest
1 tbsp. chopped parsley, fresh
1 egg
2 tsp. water

Directions:
First, make sure to place the pork chops on the counter for about 20 minutes prior to cooking to allow them to come to room temperature.

Afterwards, pat the pork dry with a paper towel, and then salt and pepper the pork to taste.

Then, beat together the egg and the 2 tsp. of water in a medium-sized bowl.

Next, stir together the grated Parmesan and the pork rinds on a large plate. Add the parsley and the garlic, and stir the mixture well.

To the side, zest a lemon, and add the zest to the plate as well, stirring well with your fingers.

Next, add each pork chop to the egg mixture, followed by the plate with the Parmesan, coating it well. Add the pork chops to the air fryer, and then cook at 400 degrees Fahrenheit for four minutes.

Afterwards, flip the pork chops and cook for an additional 6 minutes, or until the pork is browned. Note that cooking time alters based on the thickness of the pork chops.

Serve the pork warm, and enjoy.

Coconut Curry with Pork

Recipe Makes 8 Servings.
Preparation Time: 2 hours marinate time plus 25 minutes

Nutritional Information Per Serving: 296 calories, 5 grams carbohydrates, 17 grams fat, 31 grams protein.

Ingredients:

2 pounds of pork, diced into smaller pieces

1 tsp. cumin

2 tsp. coconut oil

1/2 tsp. cinnamon

1/2 tsp. chili powder

1 tsp. coriander

Sliced ginger, one inch

14 ounces coconut cream

Zest from one lime

Juice from one lime

4 minced garlic cloves

1 diced onion

1/2 tsp. sea salt

1/2 tsp. pepper

Directions:

First, add the pork to a large mixing bowl. Add the coriander, cinnamon, chili powder, and cumin at this time, and stir well. Allow the pork to marinate in the spices for two hours. You can also do this overnight, if you have the time.

Preheat the air fryer to 400 degrees Fahrenheit.

Next, add the coconut oil, coconut cream, onion, garlic, and the ginger to the mixture, and stir well. Pour this mixture into the air fryer baking dish.

Cook the curry in the air fryer at 400 degrees Fahrenheit for 17 to 20 minutes, or until the mixture is bubbly and hot and the pork is cooked all the way through.

Next, add the zest from the lime, lime juice, and the salt and pepper. Cook for an additional five minutes, and then serve the pork curry warm.

Ketogenic Air Fryer Fish Recipes

Carb Cakes with Spicy Mayonnaise

Recipe Makes 4 Servings.
Preparation Time: 15 minutes

Nutritional Information Per Serving: 163 calories, 7.5 grams carbohydrates, 11 grams protein, 8 grams fat, 1 gram fiber.

Ingredients:
1/3 cup almond flour
1 egg
10 ounces crab meat
1/3 cup diced green peppers
1/3 cup diced red peppers
1/4 cup mayonnaise
Juice from one half of a lemon
1 tsp. Old Bay seasoning
1 tsp. Worcestershire sauce
1 tsp. dry mustard powder
1/2 tsp. sea salt
1/2 tsp. pepper

Extra 1 tbsp. of almond flour for the patties

Directions:
First, preheat the air fryer to 400 degrees Fahrenheit.

To the side, stir together the almond flour, egg, crab meat, green and red peppers, mayonnaise, juice from half of a lemon, and the rest of the ingredients. Stir well, and then form the mixture into patties.

Then, dust the crab patties with the extra almond flour.

Then, place the crab patties inside the air fryer, and cook them for 10 minutes. Remove the patties from the air fryer, and allow them to cool for three minutes prior to serving.

Nourishing Shrimp Scampi

Recipe Makes 4 Servings.
Preparation Time: 15 minutes

Nutritional Information Per Serving: 261 calories, 3.3 grams carbohydrates, 14 grams fat, 26 grams protein, .3 grams fiber.

Ingredients:
1 pound shrimp, about 23 to 25 pieces, defrosted
1 tsp. dried chives
4 tbsp. ghee
1 tbsp. minced garlic
1 1/2 tbsp. lemon juice
2 tsp. red pepper flakes
1 tbsp. chopped basil
2 tbsp. white wine

Directions:

First, turn on the air fryer to 330 degrees Fahrenheit. Allow it to heat while you prep the rest of the ingredients.

Next, place the red pepper flakes, garlic, and the ghee in the six-inch pan.

Allow the mixture to cook for a full two minutes, stirring about halfway through. The ghee should melt completely.

Next, open the air fryer. Add the lemon juice, chives, basil, white wine, and then the shrimp, all in that order. Stir slowly and carefully.

Next, allow the shrimp to cook for five minutes, stirring only a single time.

After five minutes, give the mixture another stir, and remove the six-inch pan carefully, using mitts. Allow the pan to rest for 45 seconds on the countertop, ensuring that the shrimp cooks in what's left of the heat in the ghee.

Stir after 45 seconds. Serve with a sprinkling of basil, and enjoy.

Fried Catfish

Recipe Makes 4 Servings.
Preparation Time: 1 hour and 10 minutes

Nutritional Information Per Serving: 191 calories, 2.6 carbohydrates, 17 grams protein, 12 grams fat, 0.5 grams fiber.

Ingredients:
4 fillets of catfish
1 tbsp. olive oil
1/4 cup almond flour
2 tsp. garlic powder
2 tsp. onion powder
1 tsp. cayenne pepper

Directions:
First, preheat the air fryer to 400 degrees Fahrenheit for ten minutes.

While it's preheating, rinse off the fish and pat the fillets dry.

Then, add the almond flour, garlic powder, onion powder, and the cayenne pepper to a medium-sized bowl. Dredge the catfish fillets inside the powder mixture.

Next, brush each fillet of catfish with olive oil, and place the fillets in the air fryer basket.

Close the air fryer and cook the fillets for ten minutes. If you have to, you can do them in a few different batches.

After ten minutes, flip the fish and cook for an additional ten minutes. Next, flip the fish a final time, and cook for three more minutes—or until it's golden brown.

Serve the catfish fillets warm, and enjoy.

Lemon Butter Glazed Salmon

Recipe Makes 2 Servings.
Preparation Time: 16 minutes

Nutritional Information Per Serving: 394 calories, 3.6 grams carbohydrates, 35 grams protein, 23 grams fat, .5 grams fiber.

Ingredients:
2 salmon fillets
1/3 cup white wine
1/2 tsp. olive oil
1 tbsp. minced garlic

3 tbsp. lemon juice
2 tbsp. butter, salted
1 tsp. salt
1 tsp. pepper

Directions:
First, preheat the air fryer for ten minutes at 400 degrees Fahrenheit.

Next, place the salmon on the air fryer's grill pan, and cook the salmon for six minutes or until the salmon is done and flakes easily with a fork.

While the air fryer heats and the salmon cooks, stir up the lemon butter sauce. To do this, simply sauté the garlic in the olive oil for two minutes (on the stovetop). Then, add the lemon juice and the white wine, and bring the mixture to a boil.

When it begins to boil, reduce the heat to low and allow it to cook for an additional five minutes.

At this time, remove the mixture from the heat and add the butter, along with the salt and pepper. Pour the sauce over the cooked salmon, and enjoy.

Ketogenic Air Fryer Vegetarian Recipes

Vegetarian Keto "Buffalo Wings" with Cauliflower

Recipe Makes 4 Servings.
Preparation Time: 20 minutes

Nutritional Information Per Serving: 226 calories, 8.3 grams carbohydrates, 20 grams fat, 3.5 grams protein, 4 grams fiber.

Ingredients:
4 cups of chopped cauliflower florets—so that they look vaguely the size of buffalo wings
1 cup almond flour
1/3 cup ghee
1/3 cup buffalo sauce

Directions:
First, add the ghee to a microwave-able bowl and melt it in the microwave. Then, whisk the buffalo sauce with the ghee using a fork.

Next, dip the cauliflower florets into the buffalo sauce mixture, making sure to coat it well in the sauce. Then, dip the florets in with the almond flour, coating it well, and then add them to the air fryer. They don't need to be in a single layer. They can all kind of be on top of one another, and it'll still work well.

Next, air fry the cauliflower florets for 17 minutes at 350 degrees Fahrenheit, shaking the basket a few times as you go. The cauliflower florets should be golden brown.

Serve warm, and enjoy.

Broccoli and Cheese Quiche

Recipe Makes 4 Servings.
Preparation Time: 40 minutes

Nutritional Information Per Serving: 164 calories, 12 grams carbohydrates, 8 grams fat, 10 grams protein, 3.3 grams fiber.

Ingredients:
1 head of broccoli, chopped into florets
1/3 cup grated cheddar cheese
3 diced carrots
1 tomato, diced

1 tsp. dried parsley
1 tsp. dried thyme
1/3 cup chopped feta cheese
1/2 cup milk, whole
2 eggs
1/2 tsp. salt
1/2 tsp. pepper

Directions:
First, chop the broccoli and dice the carrots. Add the vegetables to the air fryer and cook at 300 degrees Fahrenheit for 10 minutes, or until they're soft.

Then, stir together the seasonings in a medium-sized dish. Add the eggs and the milk, stirring slowly until the mixture is pale but well-assimilated.

After the vegetables are finished, line a quiche dish with the vegetables, and then add the sliced tomatoes and the cheeses to the top, making sure to spread them out evenly.

Next, pour the milk and eggs mixture over the top. Add any additional cheeses, if you please.

Then, place the quiche dish into the air fryer. Cook for 20 minutes at 370 degrees Fahrenheit.

Afterwards, allow the quiche to cool for ten minutes and then serve.

Ketogenic Air Fryer Side Dish Recipes

Air Fried Brussels Sprouts

Recipe Makes 2 Servings.
Preparation Time: 15 minutes

Nutritional Information Per Serving: 100 calories, 8 grams carbohydrates, 7 grams fat, 3 grams protein, 3 grams fiber.

Ingredients:
2 cups of Brussels sprouts, chopped in half
1 tbsp. balsamic vinegar
1 tbsp. olive oil
1/2 tsp. sea salt

Directions:
First, toss together the Brussels sprouts, vinegar, salt, and the olive oil in a medium-sized bowl.

Next, air fry the Brussels sprouts for ten minutes in the air fryer, making sure to shake the basket after five minutes and then again at the eight-minute mark.

Serve the crispy Brussels sprouts warm, and enjoy.

Crispy Asparagus

Recipe Makes 4 Servings.
Preparation Time: 15 minutes

Nutritional Information Per Serving: 41 calories, 4 grams carbohydrates, 2 grams protein, 2 grams fat, 2.3 grams fiber.

Ingredients:
1/2 bunch asparagus, sliced at the two-inch mark from the bottom
1 tsp. sea salt
1 tsp. black pepper
2 tsp. olive oil

Directions:
First, add the asparagus to an air fryer basket, and spritz them with oil. Then, add black pepper and sea salt, shaking the asparagus well in the basket.

Place the basket in the air fryer and bake the asparagus at 400 degrees Fahrenheit for 10 minutes.

Afterwards, serve the asparagus warm, and enjoy.

Garlic Bread "Muffins"

Recipe Makes 12 Servings.
Preparation Time: 25 minutes

Nutritional Information Per Serving: 219 calories, 3.6 grams carbohydrates, 18 grams fat, 10 grams protein, 1 gram fiber.

Ingredients:
4 eggs, large-sized
6 minced garlic cloves
2 tsp. baking powder
1/2 cup sour cream
1 tsp. salt
3 cups almond flour
1 1/4 cup cheddar cheese, shredded
5 ounces mozzarella, shredded
1/3 cup chopped parsley, fresh
6 tbsp. melted butter

Directions:
First, preheat your air fryer to 300 degrees Fahrenheit. Make sure that whatever muffin baking pan you're using (which fits inside the air fryer) is greased with either butter or oil.

Next, melt the butter in the microwave or over the stove, and stir the butter with the garlic. Set this mixture to the side.

Next, using a blender, mix together the eggs, sour cream, and salt. Do this until the mixture is well-assimilated. Next, add the baking powder, parsley, cheddar cheese, and almond flour, and process until the mixture is completely smooth and well-mixed.

Divide this batter mixture in each of the muffin tins (or ramekins)—about halfway to the top (you won't use all of it in this step), and make a small "indent" in the center of each. Add the mozzarella into the center of the wells, and then drizzle the top of them with the garlic butter.

Next, pour the rest of the batter over the cheese, and brush the tops of the muffins with the rest of the garlic butter.

Air fry the muffins for 17 minutes, or until the muffins are golden brown. Remove them from the air fryer and allow them to cool for about ten minutes prior to serving.

Mashed "Potatoes" with Parmesan

Recipe Makes 5 Servings.
Preparation Time: 20 minutes

Nutritional Information Per Serving: 131 calories, 6.1 grams carbohydrates, 3 grams fat, 20 grams protein, 2.8 grams fiber.

Ingredients:
2 heads of cauliflower, chopped into florets
1/3 cup Parmesan cheese, grated
2 cups chicken or vegetable broth
1/3 cup chopped chives, fresh
1/2 tsp. salt
1/2 tsp. pepper

Directions:
After prepping everything, add the cauliflower and the broth to your air fryer, and give the mixture a good stir. Cook on 400 degrees Fahrenheit for 15 minutes. The cauliflower should be very tender.

Next, use a slotted spoon to remove the cauliflower from the air fryer, and place it in a blender or a food processor. Process the mixture until it's smooth.

Next, pour the pureed cauliflower to a large bowl, and stir it with the Parmesan and the chives. Add salt and pepper to taste, and serve warm.

Curried Cauliflower

Recipe Makes 4 Servings.
Preparation Time: 20 minutes

Nutritional Information Per Serving: 91 calories, 12 grams carbohydrates, 3 grams fat, 4 grams protein, 6 grams fiber.

Ingredients:
2 pounds of cauliflower, chopped into florets
2 tsp. lemon juice
1 tbsp. olive oil
2 tsp. curry powder
1 tsp. salt
2 tbsp. chopped cilantro

Directions:
First, preheat your air fryer to 400 degrees Fahrenheit.

Next, slice the cauliflower into florets, and toss them in a large bowl with the olive oil. Add the salt and the curry powder, tossing in a similar fashion to coat well.

Next, spread out the cauliflower in your air fryer, and cook it for 14 minutes, or until it begins to brown.

After it cooks, return the cauliflower to the bowl, and toss it with the lemon juice and the cilantro. Serve warm, and enjoy.

Walnut Kale with Bacon Flair

Recipe Makes 10 Servings.
Preparation Time: 40 minutes

Nutritional Information Per Serving: 166 calories, 10 grams carbohydrates, 10 grams fat, 8 grams protein, 2 grams fiber.

Ingredients:
4 slices turkey bacon, uncooked and chopped
1 cup mascarpone cheese
1/2 cup almond milk
3 minced garlic cloves
1 tbsp. butter

12 cups kale, chopped roughly
1/2 tsp. nutmeg, ground
1/2 cup grated Parmesan cheese
1/2 tsp. salt
1/2 tsp. pepper
1/3 cup chopped walnuts

Directions:
First, preheat the air fryer to 320 degrees Fahrenheit.

Next, add the bacon pieces to a skillet and cook on medium-high heat until golden. Remove the bacon to the side.

Next, add the garlic and the butter to the skillet and cook for one minute more, until you can smell the garlic.

Next, add the almond milk and the nutmeg. Stir well and cook for one minute before adding the kale, heaping it and cooking for four minutes, or until it's wilted.

At this time, add the mascarpone and the Parmesan, and stir well. Season the mixture to taste.

Then, add the mixture to a baking dish, which can fit into the air fryer.

Cook the mixture in the air fryer for 25 minutes. At this time, add the bacon and the walnuts to the top of the mixture, and allow it to air fry for an additional seven minutes.

Serve warm, and enjoy.

Buttery Bok Choy

Recipe Makes 4 Servings.
Preparation Time: 10 minutes

Nutritional Information Per Serving: 49 calories, 3.9 grams carbohydrates, 3 grams fat, 3 grams protein, 2 grams fiber.

Ingredients:
2 tbsp. water
1 tsp. sesame oil
1 tbsp. oyster sauce
1 tbsp. butter
2 tsp. soy sauce
2 heads of chopped bok choy
1 tbsp. olive oil
1/2 tsp. salt

1/2 tsp. pepper

Directions:
First, stir together the sesame oil, soy sauce, water, and oyster sauce in a medium-sized bowl and set the mixture to the side.

Next, heat the air fryer to 400 degrees Fahrenheit. Add the olive oil, bok choy and the salt and pepper, and stir, cooking, for three minutes.

Next, add the butter and the soy sauce mixture and cook for an additional five minutes, stirring occasionally, until the bok choy begins to get crispy.

Serve the bok choy warm, and enjoy.

Ketogenic Air Fryer Snacks and Appetizers

Mozzarella Sticks

Recipe Makes 10 Sticks.
Preparation Time: 50 minutes

Nutritional Information Per Serving: 67 calories, 1.1 grams carbohydrates, 6 grams protein, 4 grams fat, 0 grams fiber.

Ingredients:

5 ounces mozzarella cheese, sliced into sticks (or you could use mozzarella string cheese sticks)
1 tsp. garlic powder
3/4 cup grated Parmesan cheese
1 egg
1 tsp. Italian seasoning
1/2 tsp. salt
1/2 tsp. pepper

Directions:

First, stir together the salt, pepper, and egg in a medium-sized bowl.

To the side, stir together the garlic powder, Parmesan cheese, Italian seasoning, and the salt and pepper in a medium-sized bowl.

Next, dip the pieces of mozzarella into the egg, salt, and pepper mixture, and then dip them into the seasoning. Place the cheese sticks in a small storage container, and put them in the freezer for 30 minutes.

Preheat the air fryer to 400 degrees Fahrenheit, making sure it preheats for ten minutes before cooking.

Add the mozzarella sticks to the air fryer basket and allow them to cook for 8 minutes, or until they're golden brown. Serve the mozzarella sticks warm, and enjoy.

Zucchini Fries for All

Recipe Makes 4 Servings.
Preparation Time: 15 minutes

Nutritional Information Per Serving: 101 calories, 4.5 grams carbohydrates, 9 grams protein, 5 grams fat, 1.2 grams fiber.

Ingredients:

2 zucchinis, large-sized
1 egg
1 cup grated Parmesan cheese
1/2 tsp. black pepper
1/2 tsp. garlic powder

Directions:
First, preheat the air fryer to 400 degrees Fahrenheit.

Next, slice the zucchini in half, from top to bottom, four times each. This will produce eight long zucchini fries. Then, you should slice the zucchini fries once in half, so that you have about sixteen zucchini fries in total.

Next, crack the egg into one bowl, and whisk it with your fork. Stir together the garlic powder, the Parmesan cheese, and the black pepper in a separate bowl, and stir well.

Add each zucchini fry to the egg mixture, then dunk it in the spice mixture. Set each fry to the side as you prep the others.

Next, add the zucchini fries to the air fryer. You'll probably only be able to do them in half batches. Cook them in the air fryer for about ten minutes, or until golden brown. Then, remove them and fry up the second batch.

Serve the fries warm, and enjoy.

Air Fried Jalapeno Rings

Recipe Makes 4 Servings.
Preparation Time: 10 minutes

Nutritional Information Per Serving: 20 calories, 1 gram carbohydrate, 1 gram protein, 1 gram fat, .2 grams fiber.

Ingredients:
1 large jalapeno, sliced
1/2 tsp. onion powder
1/2 tsp. garlic powder
1/2 tsp. Cajun seasoning
1/2 tsp. salt
1/2 tsp. pepper
1 egg

Directions:
First, preheat the air fryer to 400 degrees Fahrenheit.

Stir together the onion powder, garlic powder, Cajun seasoning, salt, and pepper in a medium-sized bowl.

Crack the egg into a separate medium-sized bowl.

Next, dip the jalapeño pieces into the egg, and drop the jalapeños into the spice mixture immediately after, coating them.

Next, add the jalapeños to the air fryer, making sure to make only a single layer. Cook the jalapeños in the air fryer until they're crispy, turning them over a single time.

The amount of time will vary depending on how big your jalapeños are. Serve warm, and enjoy.

Avocado Fries

Recipe Makes 4 Servings.
Preparation Time: 20 minutes

Nutritional Information Per Serving: 131 calories, 5 grams carbohydrates, 12 grams fat, 2 grams protein, 3.8 grams fiber.

Ingredients:
½ tsp. salt

½ cup almond flour

1 avocado, sliced and pitted and peeled

½ egg

Directions:

First, toss together the almond flour and the salt in a small bowl.

Crack half an egg into a bowl and whisk it. Then, dredge your avocado slices in with the egg, and place them in the almond flour so that they're well-coated.

Next, place the slices of avocado in a single layer in the air fryer's basket. Make sure none of the avocado 'fries' overlap one another.

Next, air fry the avocado 'fries' for ten minutes at 400 degrees Fahrenheit. At around the five minute mark, make sure you shake the air fryer basket vigorously, so that you flip the fries over.

Afterwards, serve the avocado fries warm, and enjoy.

Crunchy Kale Chips

Recipe Makes 4 Servings.

Preparation Time: 10 minutes

Nutritional Information Per Serving: 115 calories, 10 grams carbohydrates, 3.8 grams protein, 7 grams fat, 2 grams fiber.

Ingredients:
5 cups of kale, packed, with the stems taken off
1 tsp. onion powder
1 tsp. garlic powder
2 tbsp. olive oil
1/2 tsp. salt
1 tbsp. nutritional yeast flakes

Directions:
First, toss the kale pieces with the onion powder, garlic powder, olive oil, salt, and the nutritional yeast flakes. Then, dump the kale into the air fryer's basket.

Cook the kale chips in the air fryer at 375 degrees Fahrenheit for five minutes. Make sure to shake the basket after two minutes.

Serve warm and crispy, and enjoy.

Ketogenic Air Fryer Dessert Recipes

Ketogenic Cream Cheese Cookies in the Air Fryer

Recipe Makes 15 Cookies.
Preparation Time: 10 minutes

Nutritional Information Per Serving: 85 calories, 6 grams carbohydrates, 7 grams fat, 1 gram protein, 1.6 gram fiber.

Ingredients:
1/2 cup butter
3/4 cup coconut flour
1 egg
4 tbsp. cream cheese, softened
1/2 cup Erythritol
1/2 tsp. baking powder
1/2 tsp. salt
1 tsp. vanilla

Directions:
First, in a medium-sized bowl, stir together the erythritol and the cream cheese. Add the softened butter, and stir well.

Next, add the egg and the vanilla, and beat until the mixture is completely smooth.

Next, add the baking powder, coconut flour, and the salt and stir well until the mixture is sticky and well-assimilated.

Next, preheat the air fryer to 350 degrees Fahrenheit. Form the cookies into small balls and place them on the baking sheet within the air fryer. Allow the cookies to cook for six minutes, or until they're golden brown on the top.

Remove the cookies from the air fryer and either serve warm or hot.

Low Carb Macaroons

Recipe Makes 10 Cookies.
Preparation Time: 15 minutes

Nutritional Information Per Serving: 67 calories, 3 grams carbohydrates, 5 grams fat, 2 grams protein, 1 gram fiber.

Ingredients:

3/4 cup coconut, shredded
1/3 cup almond flour
3 eggs, just the whites
1 tbsp. vanilla
1 tbsp. coconut oil
2 tbsp. agave nectar

Directions:
First, stir together the coconut and the almond flour in a medium-sized bowl.

Next, melt the coconut oil over the stove. When it's melted, add the agave nectar, and stir well.

Place a medium-sized bowl in the freezer. You'll need this to be chilly for the egg whites.

Next, add the agave and coconut oil to the almond flour mixture and stir well.

Afterwards, add the egg whites to the freezer-prepped bowl, and whisk them until they're very foamy and stiff, using either a whisk or your fork.

Next, add the egg whites to the almond flour mixture, ensuring that you don't stir too quickly or over-mix. Make sure you keep some of the "fluffiness" from the egg whites.

Next, spoon out ten to twelve cookies onto your baking sheet, and place the baking sheet in the air fryer.

Air fry the cookies at 350 degrees Fahrenheit for six minutes, or until they're browned at the top.

Remove the cookies from the fryer at this time, and ensure they cool prior to removing them from the baking sheet.

Ketogenic Cheesecake with Blueberries

Recipe Makes 8 Servings.
Preparation Time: 20 minutes

Nutritional Information Per Serving: 207 calories, 4 grams carbohydrates, 4 grams protein, 19 grams fat, 0.5 gram fiber.

Ingredients:
5 eggs
1 stick of butter
1/2 tsp. baking powder
1/2 cup cream cheese, cubed
4 tbsp. agave nectar
2 tsp. vanilla

1/2 cup blueberries

Directions:
First, add the stick of butter, eggs, baking powder, cream cheese, agave nectar, and the vanilla together in a medium-sized mixing bowl. Mix together the ingredients using a stick blender, doing so until it's smooth.

Next, pour the mixture into a baking dish (one that can fit inside your air fryer).

Then, drop the blueberries into the cream cheese mixture, doing it so that they're spread over the mixture.

Bake the cheesecake in the air fryer for 15 minutes at 300 degrees Fahrenheit. Make sure the cheesecake is cooked in the center.

Then, allow the mixture to cool prior to slicing and serving.

Ketogenic Brownies

Recipe Makes 12 Servings.

Preparation Time: 15 minutes

Nutritional Information Per Serving: 202 calories, 7 grams carbohydrates, 5 grams protein, 18 grams fat, 2.3 grams fiber.

Ingredients:
1 1/2 sticks of melted butter

6 eggs

2 tsp. vanilla

1 cup cocoa, unsweetened

½ tsp. baking powder

5 ounces cream cheese, fully softened

4 tbsp. agave nectar

Directions:
First, add the butter, eggs, vanilla, baking powder, cream cheese, agave nectar, and cocoa to a medium-sized mixing bowl. Use a stick blender to blend the ingredients until smooth.

Then, add the mixture to a baking dish and place the dish in the air fryer. Bake the brownies for 15 minutes at 300 degrees Fahrenheit, or until it's completely cooked in the center.

Slice the brownies into squares, and serve.

Peanut Butter Cookies

Recipe Makes 12 Cookies.
Preparation Time: 10 minutes

Nutritional Information: 78 calories, 4.8 grams carbohydrates, 3 grams protein, 6 grams fat, 0.7 grams fiber.

Ingredients:
1/2 cup peanut butter, creamy
1/4 tsp. baking soda
1/8 cup agave nectar
1 tsp. honey
1/2 egg
1/8 cup dark chocolate chips

Directions:
First, stir together the peanut butter, baking soda, honey, agave nectar, and the half an egg, making sure to mix until very smooth—even using a hand mixer, if that's an option.

Then, add the chocolate chips, and give the mixture a good stir.

Next, roll the dough into individual cookies and place them on the baking sheet. Press on the dough with a fork in first one direction, then the other—the way peanut butter cookies are traditionally made.

Then, place the baking dish in the air fryer and air fry them for 7 minutes at 300 degrees Fahrenheit, or until the cookies begin to brown.

Remove the cookies from the air fryer and allow them to cook prior to serving.

Individual Chocolate and Peanut Butter Cake

Recipe Makes 2 Servings.
Preparation Time: 10 minutes

Nutritional Information Per Serving:161 calories, 11 grams carbohydrates, 5 grams protein, 11 grams fat, 2 grams fiber.

Ingredients:
2 tbsp. agave nectar
1 tbsp. cocoa powder, unsweetened
1/2 tsp. vanilla
1 tbsp. heavy cream
1 egg
1 tsp. butter, salted and melted

1/4 tsp. baking powder

1 tbsp. peanut butter

Directions:

First, stir together the agave nectar, baking powder, vanilla, and the cocoa powder. When well assimilated, add the heavy cream, and the egg, stirring until the mixture is completely assimilated.

Melt the butter in the microwave or on the stove, and stir that in as well, mixing until completely combined.

Next, pour the cake mixture into a ramekin. Place the ramekin in the air fryer, and bake on 350 degrees Fahrenheit for four minutes.

Afterwards, melt the peanut butter in the microwave, and drizzle the peanut butter over the cake prior to serving.

Part 2

Introduction

Keto diet is a high fat, low carb diet that can transform your body into a fat-burning device. The diet of the keto is brief for a ketogenic diet. Ketogenic diets provide an appropriate diet of protein intake, an elevated level of fat and a small intake of carbohydrates. It was developed in the first place as a unique diet to control the signs of epilepsy in children. Daily meals give sufficient protein to ensure growth and repair under this diet. The calories are measured and provided in enough quantities to maintain the right weight and height for the child.

The keto diet transforms how your body metabolizes food into energy. Naturally, your body transforms carbohydrates (imagine pasta and bread) into energy glucose. Eating lots of fat and few carbs bring you in ketosis, a metabolic condition where your body releases fat rather than carbs for fuel.

How the Diet Works

The ketogenic diet pushes the body into a stage of ketosis. The body tends primarily to use carbohydrates as energy sources. The reason is that carbohydrates can be easily digested and absorbed. When the body is without carbohydrates, fats and proteins are used. Essentially, the body hierarchically uses energy. First, while it is available, the body uses carbohydrates. As a next alternative source, the body moves into fats. The last stage, usually in extreme deprivation of carbohydrates and fatty stores, is protein conversion into energy. The digestion of proteins leads to loss of muscle, as the body digests the muscle proteins.

Generally, the body enters a process of ketosis. It takes place during the fasting period. One example of this is during sleep. When the body rebuilds and expands through sleep it continues to burn fats for energy.

Carbohydrates constitute most calories in an ordinary average meal. The body carbohydrates are used as energy and other nutrients (i.e., fats and proteins) are stored Many calories in the ketogenic diet are composed of fats instead of carbohydrates. In a ketogenic diet, carbohydrate is very small and is used instantly. There is an obvious energy deficit due to the low intake of carbohydrates. The body turns to the fats it has accumulated. This switches to a fat burner from a carbohydrate user. The fats in the recently devoured meal are not instantly used; instead, they are saved for the next round. The fats of the recent meal are used as energy sources for fat-burning, and some are left to be preserved. Therefore, in order to provide the immediate energy required, the Ketogenic diet must have a high fat intake and still have a portion of the stock. Stored fat is extremely important so that the body does not absorb the protein in the muscles at fasting times.

In addition, these cycles are common in a series of days. Fasting periods occur in between meals and sleep. During these times the body also needs a constant energy supply. Protein in the muscles is next in line as the source of energy if no stored fat is present. Your diet needs to be high in fat in order to prevent this

Ketogenic diets are mainly designed to imitate starvation mode. This decreases calories and significantly eliminates carbohydrates, thus depriving the body of carbohydrates instantly and quickly converted. This compels the body to shift to the mode which consumes fat. It also induces the secretion of catecholamines (fat mobilizing hormones), cortisol (break-down and metabolic hormones) and growth hormones. This triad of hormones triggers the state of ketosis or a fat burn.

Foods to Avoid in Keto

All grains, products made from grain and potatoes

These involve wheat, rye, peas, corn, barley, millet, bulgur, sorghum, rice, amaranth, buckwheat, sprouted plant, quinoa, pasta, toast, pizza, biscuits, crackers, etc.

Both products rich in starch and sugar

These involve pies, biscuits, ice cream, agave syrup, tea, tropical fruit and the most high-sugar berries, dried fruit, cocktails, sugary soft drinks, food, etc.

All processed, inflammatory fats

It covers margarine, olive oil, soya oil, etc.

Processed goods, including soya

It is particularly crucial if you have hormone disorders.

Goods called 'low-fat' and 'low-carb'

These also involve secret sugars and other undesirable ingredients.

Farm farmed pork and non-organic farmed shrimp.

Alcohol, except for low-carbon options

Alcohol can be stopped for weight reduction as it increases hunger and is rich in calories.

1.4 Nutrient and Mineral Consumption Factors

Carbohydrates at The Keto Diet

For ketogenic diets, aim at no more than 50 grams of total carbohydrate (20 to 30 grams of net carbohydrate) per day, mostly from non-starchy vegetables, avocados and nuts. Everyone tolerates a very different amount of starch, so you're going to have to figure out what is better for you. Dropping all carbohydrates from the diet is excessive and does not contribute to an improved loss of weight.

Don't be obsessive about your ketone levels. Ketone rates will inform you how much "food" you have in your "box," but not how much food the body uses for electricity. Keto-adapted people are more prone to have lower ketone rates, mainly because their bodies may handle them more effectively than non-keto-adapted people.

Protein On a Diet of Keto

Keep your protein moderate at 0.6 to 1 gram per pound (1.3 to 2.2 grams per kilogram) of lean weight following a keto diet. For most instances, this turns into 65 to 80 grams of protein a day, often even more. The exact amount depends on gender, lean weight and level of activity. Ensure sure you're getting plenty and don't think over the protein consumption. Eating a bit extra nutrition does not slow down the weight loss. Know, protein is the most concentrated macronutrient;

it can make you feel less hungry and consume fewer calories.

If the weight loss ends on a keto diet, it certainly doesn't have any fat. Try to eat a little more protein because it suppresses your appetite, increases your metabolic rate, and helps maintain muscle mass.

The concern in specific keto diets is that excessive protein consumption contributes to gluconeogenesis, a mechanism through which the liver produces glucose from amino acids and other compounds. For certain instances, protein is a self-limiting food, which ensures that it is impossible to overeat, at least daily.

Reconsider once If you are insulin resistant or diabetic, or if you are in a state of health, be aware that not all protein sources are equal. Please consult your doctor.

Fat On a Diet of Keto

If you eat a ketogenic diet, using fat as a buffer to feed your hunger while holding your carbohydrates minimal. Remember that you do not need to monitor your fat consumption and count calories, but it can help you hit the plateau, particularly as you get close to your goal weight. If you're looking for your ideal calorie intake. Including monitoring calories, protein, fat, and electrolytes, the software contains thousands of low-carb recipes to motivate the Keto to live.

Important Hacks and Factors to Be Remembered

You may feel headaches, nausea, exhaustion, brain fog, muscle weakness, cramps, and heart palpitations during the initial phase of the ketogenic diet. Don't panic, man. "Keto Flu" is the standard treatment. I've experienced most of the symptoms myself, and if you're not prepared for it, you may be scared by these symptoms.

To minimize or even avoid the symptoms of keto flu, eat plenty of electrolyte-rich foods such as avocados, salmon and spinach. Be sure to keep yourself hydrated. Use salt and, if necessary, include magnesium supplements. (Note: Consult your doctor before taking magnesium supplements if you have kidney disease or are taking medication for high blood pressure.) If you exercise, you may feel tired, so don't push yourself too much.

The explanation of why one has been willing to adopt a low-carb diet for almost ten years is because they are striving to make things as straightforward and realistic as possible. Here are some of the strategies that often work:

Prepare your meals

Reserve time every week to prepare basics for the pantry. It's worth it. Or go one step further and make all your meals one day and then refrigerate or freeze for later.

Prepare your meals, please. To keep preparing simple, stick to recipes that need fewer ingredients and fewer hands-on time. That's what I've been working on while making recipes for this novel.

Create a compilation of them

The collection of shopping is a must. It's going to save you time and energy. Don't go shopping, too, when you're hungry. Order most of your grocery stores online, and you'll eventually find it easier to focus on what's needed.

Prep the rest of it. Was there no room to cook? Most of the recipes discussed in the book will take less than thirty minutes to prepare. Plus, they 're easy to scale. Choose two or three separate meals and double or triple the amount to provide plenty for the entire week.

The variation

Make simple changes to the recipes to make a whole new meal. Swap oils and seasoning with other flavorings. Or change the protein and use different low-carb vegetables. It's so easy.

Stay on the basics

To make cooking easier, store frozen vegetables and berries, essential pantry, condiments, canned fatty fish, nuts and seeds.

Say yes to the useful tools. Use a microwave, a pressure cooker or a slow cooker to reduce your cooking time. Each week, try to create an incredible chicken stock in my electric pressure cooker.

Stay imaginative

Turn the meat from dinner last night to lunch tomorrow. They are using the milky plants and mushrooms to create a quick frittata (shown here). The leftover herbs and even the leafy greens are perfect for making Simple Pesto and using extra egg yolks to produce Dutch sauce, Creamy Breakfast Hot Chocolate or Long-lasting Mayonnaise.

Dinning out

Eating on a ketogenic diet is even more straightforward than you would imagine. Here are a few tactics that will set you up for success:

Prepare for time. Many restaurants are uploading their menus online. If the plan is not accessible in advance, inquire for a gluten-free version and search for the right keto choices.

Avoid all high-carb foods and watch out for hidden carbs. Choose dishes that are quickly cooked, without sauces. Opt for grilled, fried, steamed or roasted meat, poultry, seafood, non-starchy vegetables or salads.

Double the order of non-starchy veg sides. Ask for keto salad dressing or extra virgin olive oil, lemon wedges and vinegar (go easy on balsamic as it is relatively high in carbs).

Still or carbonated water is always a safe choice, just like coffee or tea. Fresh-squeezed lemon or lime will jazz the water or the soda club. Opt for distilled spirits, dry wine and low-carbon cider and beer (with gluten-free options available).

Easy Low Carb Swaps

Pasta: zucchini noodles, shirataki noodles or kelp noodles;

Rice: cauli rice or shirataki rice

Roasted potatoes: Rotabaga ham, turnips, radishes or cauliflower

Potato mash: **flower mash**

Soy sauce: coconut amino or tamari sauce

Milk: Unsweetened almond or coconut milk

Rice, bulgur, and quinoa: cauli-rice or hemp seeds

Crackers: Cheese Crickets, linseed crackers, celery sticks, cucumber slices, radishes or sliced bell peppers; dehydrated vegetables; and beef chickpeas.

Sandwich: Three-minute Keto Sandwich; lettuce leaves to cover burger buns;

Tortillas: leaves of lettuce orchard

Pizza: Pizza Crust Protein

Oats and cereals: chia seeds, nuts, coconut kernels, hemp seeds

High-carbon alcoholic drinks (cocktails, gin, blenders): dry martini, vodka, club soda, dry white and red wines, prosecco, champagne, low-carbon cider and gin (gluten-free alternatives are available).

Sweeter Swaps

One tablespoon of sugar = 2 to 3 drops of liquid stevia or monk fruit OR a touch of pure powdered stevia or monk fruit OR 1 teaspoon of erythritol or swerve

One tablespoon (10 g/0.4 oz.) of sugar = 6 to 9 drops of liquid stevia or monk fruit OR 1/4 teaspoon of pure powdered stevia or monk fruit OR 1 tablespoon of erythritol or Swerve

1 cup (200 g/7.1 oz.) table (granulated) sugar = 1 cup (200 g/7.1 oz.) granulated Swerve OR 11/3 cups (267 g/9.4 oz.) granulated erythritol OR 1 cup (200 g/7.1 oz.) granulated stevia or monk fruit blend OR 1 teaspoon of pure powdered stevia or monk fruit OR 1 teaspoon of liquid stevia or liquid monk fruit

1 cup (160 g/5.6 oz.) Confectioners' Sugar = 1 cup (160 g/5.6 oz.) Confectioners' Swerve OR 1 1/3 cups (213 g/17.5 oz.) Erythritol Confectioners' (powdered)

One tablespoon (15 ml) of sugar, blackstrap or maple syrup = two teaspoons (30 ml) of yacon syrup

Easy substitutions for cooking

One clove of fresh garlic = around 1/2 teaspoon of minced garlic > half teaspoon of garlic flakes or 1/4 teaspoon of granulated garlic or 1/8 teaspoon of garlic powder

One medium onion = around 1/3 cup (70 g/2.5 oz.) of chopped onion > 1 teaspoon of onion powder or one tablespoon (5 g/0.2 oz.) of dried onion flakes

One tablespoon (15 ml) of lime juice > 1 tablespoon (15 ml) of lemon juice or 1/2 tablespoon (8 ml) of apple cider vinegar or wine vinegar

1 tsp of baking powder > 1/2 tsp of tartar cream + 1/2 tsp of baking soda OR 1/2 tsp of lemon juice + 1/2 tsp of baking soda

1 tablespoon (6 g/0.2 oz.) of freshly ground ginger / turmeric > 1/4 teaspoon of ginger powder / turmeric powder

One tablespoon of freshly chopped herbs > 1 teaspoon of dried herbs

Bone broth = beef stock, chicken stock, vegetable stock (same quantity)

Chapter 1: Air Fryer

Air fryer is a high-powered counter-top oven that fries foods by circulating superheated air around the food at high speed. Foods fried with air fryer are touted to be healthier than the deep fried counterpart because it requires less oil to produce same taste and texture in a lighter, quicker way.

Air fryer works by blowing hot air around the food in the basket to produce a crispy exterior through caramelization and mailard reactions. Mailard reaction is a kind of chemical reaction that occurs between amino acid and reducing sugars to produce browning effect in food. So long as the temperature is between 280-330°F, your meat, chips, chicken, pastries will turn brown whenever it is cook in Air Fryer.

Benefits of Keto Air Fryer

Air Fryer is health-friendly: several healthy recipes do not include fats. And the few that do, just add a few teaspoons for flavour. The food might melt off when the oil in the food is much, and the appliance may produce smoke too.

High safety standards, great for green Cooks: the system is nothing like a stove or deep frying in a pan. It's closed and eliminates the risk of having a pan full of boiling oil falling off the stove. Again, with the fryer closed, there's no risk of getting your fingers burnt or splashing hot liquid on you while the food cooks.

Most Air Fryers come with automatic cooking functions, so no need for speculations: with just a push of a button you one can cook tater tots, French fries, chicken fingers, and other foods, depending on the model you're using. The fryer regulates the temperature and the duration of cooking the foods.

Clean-up couldn't get any easier: air fryers are designed with non-stick materials, making the cleaning process really easy. With soap, water, and a nonabrasive sponge you're good to go. Soak it for a short time if there're food particles that got burned onto the basket. Cleaning the appliance with a damp sponge or paper towel works just fine too. So now that saves you the stress of disposing cups of oil after frying.

It's more convenient cooking with one appliance: cooking with the air fryers affords you so much flexibility. You can safely attend to other chores in the kitchen while your food cooks. This can be the only appliance you'll need if you've got a small kitchen.

Hacks for Your Air Fryer

Air fryers are totally exciting. They are not bulky in size as compared to regular kitchen appliances. They are also healthy and make cooking fun. Here're a few hacks to help you master usage:

Never Overload the Air Fryer

Make sure there's sufficient space in the air fryer for air flow. Since it uses cooking foods, it is important to leave some space between food to ensure proper cooking and crisping of meals. You won't get crispy foods if the air fryer is overloaded.

Mixing Intermittently

Oil helps in binding and mixing food particles when cooking, but unlike other cooking appliances that use oil, the air fryer doesn't. hence, it takes extra help to mix food properly while cooking. It's good practice to stir and mix your food for at least twice while cooking. Stir evenly halfway during cooking. If you had set the fryer's timer at 12 minutes then it should be paused at 6 minutes, that's half the cooking time to stir the food before resuming. You may also shake the air fryer from time to time to ensure proper cooking.

Maintenance

Every electrical appliance in the kitchen should be well maintained and that includes the air fryer. Clean up the air fryer twice a month at least to get rid of any unpleasant odour. If your model has a detachable fryer basket, you can wash it in a dishwater, provided it's dishwasher safe.

Maintain the Room Temperature

Fresh foods should be at room temperature before cooking to get crisper foods in lesser cooking time.

Oil/Cooking Spray

Well, in the end, even air fryers need a little greasing for maintain. Use a little cooking spray or smear some oil on the inside to prevent foods from sticking to the basket base or the fryer basket. Besides, meals a bit tastier with a little amount of oil.

Warm Up the Air Fryer First

Most times its best to preheat the air fryer before using it. Be sure to check and follow through the recipe procedures. Preheating the air fryer ensures it's hot enough to make your food get really crispy.

Beyond Frying

It's not just all about frying alone. The air fryer can be used as a fan oven to make lasagna, cook pizza, noodles, and lot more. Check the manual and discover other amazing recipes you can fix with the air fryer in your kitchen.

How to Cook with an Air Fryer

When your new appliance arrives at your doorstep, take it out of the box and dismantle it.

- Take out removable parts like the tray and basket.
- Wash them well and let them dry well before use.
- When ready to start cooking, re-assemble and place it on a flat, heat-resistant surface, at least eight inches away from the wall
- Plug it to electric source and power it on
- Let it run for 10 minutes without any food, this allows it to gas-off (check your manufacturers manual for advice on first time use)
- You may lightly grease the basket with oil
- Also toss the food you plan to fry with little oil and carefully arrange into the basket
- Set the temperature and time according to recipe instructions

How to Clean your Air Fryer

Cooking is fun, but cleaning is not something anyone looks forward to. Though cleaning up after cooking can be a deal breaker, it's something you can't run away from. But cleaning your air fryer is simple. To clean your air fryer:

• Read your manufacturers manual for specific instructions on how to clean your model of Air fryer.

• Make sure any materials required for cleaning are available, like a soft bristle brush, a non-abrasive sponge, a cotton or microfiber cloth, and dish soap.

• Before you start cleaning your machine, unplug it from power source and give it about 15 to 25 minutes to cool.

• Using a damp cloth, properly wipe the outside parts of your Air fryer, removing any grease or food bits.

• Using soap and warm water, wipe the inside parts of your machine.

• To easily clean the heating element, turn your Air fryer upside down and wipe the bottom with a non-abrasive sponge.

• To clean up any dried and stubborn food residues, use baking soda. Mix it with little water to form a paste, apply it to a sponge, and use it to scrub the dirty surface. Then wipe clean with a damp cloth.

• Sometimes food bits may stick on the basket or baking pan. Let them soak for some minutes before cleaning.

How to Get the Most out of Your Air Fryer

• Lightly coat the basket with oil to prevent food from sticking on it.

• Toss ingredients with additional oil to help them crisp beautifully. (Most fatty foods will not require extra oil to crisp.)

• Avoid overcrowding your basket so that your food browns and crisps evenly

• If your ingredients can't fit into the basket, cook in several batches.

• Overcrowding the basket will also make your food take longer to cook.

• Turn your food using a pair of tongs half-way through cooking to allow even distribution of heat.

• Air fryers are not a set-and-forget kind of appliance. You can pull out the basket anytime to monitor how the cooking is going.

• Put some bread or water at the bottom to prevent it from smoking. Drippings from the food collects at the bottom and can smoke if there is nothing to soak it up.

• Light ingredients may be blown into the fan and can cause problems.

• Line the basket with parchment paper to ease the clean-up process.

Troubleshooting your Air Fryer

Cooking Problem

<u>My food is very soggy, dry, or chewy</u>:

The solution is to apply a coating of oil to achieve the best results and make sure to follow every recipe for air frying exactly as it is written.

Power Supply Issues

<u>My air fryer isn't getting any power, even if it's switched on</u>

The solution is to see if everything is connected properly and their fuses are all running. Then, check out the timer and make sure it's not set yet, because sometimes air fryers don't start if the timer is still, running. If none of these are working, replace your air fryer or get it fixed if possible.

White Smoke

<u>There is white smoke coming out from my fryer</u>

White smoke indicates that there is too much fat in the food items that are being cooked. Though, it's not harmful; it's irritating nonetheless. Make sure that you have added some water to the bottom drawer to stop the grease from overheating. Also, make sure you put less fatty foods in the air fryer to cook.

Black Smoke

<u>Black smoke emerging out of your air fryer</u>

It can be a more alarming issue compared to the white one. Unplug the unit immediately if you do observe such behavior. Black smoke emerging out of your air fryer can prove to a more alarming issue compared to the white one. Black smoke may result from burnt food. Make sure you cleaned the air fryer properly from its previous use. Clumsy cleaning can mean that some food ended up stuck to the air fryer's heater, and is now burnt. Turn the machine off, let it cool down completely, and then check if there is any food left in the heater.

It can also be caused when the circuit may have got faulty or the heating element has been damaged. Take it to repair center certified to fix your specific model.

Chapter 2. Breakfast Recipes

1. Breakfast Liver Pate

Preparation   time: **5**   **minutes**
Cooking   time: **10**   **minutes**
Servings: **7**

Ingredients:

1 lb. chicken liver

1 teaspoon salt

½ teaspoon cilantro, dried

1 yellow onion, diced

1 teaspoon ground black pepper

1 cup water

4 tablespoons butter

Directions:

Chop the chicken liver roughly and place it in the air fryer basket tray. Add water to air fryer basket tray and add diced onion. Preheat your air fryer to 360°Fahrenheit and cook chicken liver for 10-minutes. When it is finished cooking, drain the chicken liver. Transfer the chicken liver to blender, add butter, ground black pepper and dried cilantro and blend. Once you get a pate texture, transfer to liver pate bowl and serve immediately or keep in the fridge for later.

*Nutrition: **calories 173, fat 10.8, fiber 5, carbs 2.2, protein 16.1***

2. Breakfast Meatloaf Slices

Preparation time: **10** minutes
Cooking time: **20** minutes
Servings: **6**

Ingredients:

8-ounces ground pork
7-ounces ground beef
1 teaspoon olive oil
1 teaspoon butter
1 tablespoon oregano, dried
1 teaspoon cayenne pepper
1 teaspoon salt
1 tablespoon chives
1 tablespoon almond flour
1 egg
1 onion, diced

Directions:

Beat egg in a bowl. Add the ground beef and ground pork. Add the chives, almond flour, cayenne pepper, salt, dried oregano, and butter. Add diced onion to ground beef mixture. Use hands to shape a meatloaf mixture.

Preheat the air fryer to 350°Fahrenheit. Spray the inside of the air fryer basket with olive oil and place the meatloaf inside it. Cook the meatloaf for 20-minutes.

When the meatloaf has cooked, allow it to chill for a bit. Slice and serve it.

Nutrition: ***calories 176, fat 6.2, carbs 3.4, protein 22.2***

3. No-Bun Breakfast Bacon Burger

Preparation time: **10** minutes
Cooking time: **8** minutes
Servings: **2**
Ingredients:
8-ounces ground beef
2-ounces lettuce leaves
½ teaspoon minced garlic
1 teaspoon olive oil
½ teaspoon sea salt
1 teaspoon ground black pepper
1 teaspoon butter
4-ounces bacon, cooked
1 egg
½ yellow onion, diced
½ cucumber, slice finely
½ tomato, slice finely
Directions:

Begin by whisking the egg in a bowl, then add the ground beef and combine well. Add cooked, chopped bacon to the ground beef mixture. Add butter, ground black pepper, minced garlic, and salt. Mix and make burgers.

Preheat your air fryer to 370°Fahrenheit. Spray the air fryer basket with olive oil and place the burgers inside of it.

Cook the burgers for 8-minutes on each side. Meanwhile, slice the cucumber, onion, and tomato finely. Place the tomato, onion, and cucumber onto the lettuce leaves. When the burgers are cooked, allow them to chill at room temperature, and place them over the vegetables and serve.

*Nutrition: **calories 618, fat 37.8, carbs 8.6, protein 59.4***

4. Minced Beef Keto Breakfast Sandwich

Preparation time: **10** minutes
Cooking time: **16** minutes
Servings: **2**

Ingredients:

6-ounces minced beef

4 lettuce leaves

1 teaspoon flax seeds

1 teaspoon olive oil

½ teaspoon ground black pepper

½ teaspoon chili flakes

½ tomato, sliced

½ avocado, pitted, sliced

Directions:

Combine the chili flakes with the minced beef and salt. Add the flax seeds and stir the meat mixture using a fork. Preheat your air fryer to 370°Fahrenheit. Pour the olive oil into the air fryer basket tray.

Make 2 burgers from the beef mixture and place them in the air fryer basket. Cook the burgers for 8-minutes on each side. Meanwhile, slice the avocado and tomato. Place the avocado and tomato onto 2 lettuce leaves.

Add the cooked minced beef burgers and serve them hot!

Nutrition: ***calories 292, fat 12, fiber 17.9, carbs 5.9, protein 27.2***

5. Breakfast Beef Chili

Preparation	time:	**10**	minutes
Cooking	time:	**10**	minutes

Servings: **4**

Ingredients:

8-ounces ground beef

½ yellow onion, diced

1 teaspoon tomato puree

6-ounces cheddar cheese, shredded

1 teaspoon parsley, dried

1 teaspoon cilantro, dried

1 teaspoon oregano, dried

1 tablespoon dill weed

1 teaspoon mustard

1 tablespoon butter

Directions:

Combine ground beef with diced onion in a bowl. Sprinkle the mixture with tomato puree, cilantro, parsley, oregano and dried dill. Then add the butter and mustard and mix well. Preheat your air fryer to 380°Fahrenheit. Add ground beef mixture to air fryer basket tray and cook the chili for 9-minutes. After about 6-minutes of cooking stir the chili. When the chili is cooked, sprinkle the top with shredded cheddar cheese and stir carefully. Transfer chili mixture into serving bowls. Serve warm.

Nutrition: calories 315, fat 20.8, fiber 5, carbs 2.9, protein 28.4

6. Baked Eggs & Sausage Muffins

Preparation   time: **10**   **minutes**
Cooking   time: **20**   **minutes**
Servings: **2**

Ingredients:

3 eggs
¼ cup cream
2 sausages, boiled
Chopped fresh herbs
Sea salt to taste
4 tablespoons cheese, grated
1 piece of bread, sliced lengthwise

Directions:

Preheat your air fryer to 360°Fahrenheit. Break the eggs in a bowl, add cream, and scramble. Grease 3 muffin cups with cooking spray. Add equal amounts of egg mixture into each. Arrange sliced sausages and bread slices into muffin cups, sinking into egg mixture. Sprinkle the tops with cheese, and salt to taste. Cook the muffins for 20-minutes. Season with fresh herbs and serve warm.

Nutrition: calories 242, fat 12.5, carbs 10.2, protein 14.3

7. Spinach & Parsley Baked Omelet

Preparation	time:	**10**	minutes
Cooking	time:	**10**	minutes

Servings: **1**

Ingredients:

1 teaspoon olive oil

3 eggs

3 tablespoons ricotta cheese

1 tablespoon parsley, chopped

¼ cup spinach, chopped

Salt and pepper to taste

Directions:

Preheat your air fryer to 330°Fahrenheit. Whisk eggs adding salt and pepper as seasoning. Heat the olive oil in air fryer. Stir in the ricotta, spinach, and parsley with eggs. Pour the egg mixture into baking dish and cook in air fryer for 10-minutes. Serve warm.

Nutrition: calories 235, fat 9.2, carbs 8.4, protein 11.6

8. English Breakfast

Preparation time: **10** minutes
Cooking time: **20** minutes
Servings: **4**

Ingredients:

8 medium sausages

8 slices of back bacon

4 eggs

8 slices of toast

1 can baked beans

2 tomatoes, sliced, sautė

½ cup mushrooms, finely sliced, sautė

1 tablespoon olive oil

Directions:

Preheat your air fryer to 320°Fahrenheit. Heat olive oil in saucepan over medium-high heat. Add mushrooms to pan and sautė for a few minutes. Remove mushrooms from pan and set aside, add tomatoes to pan and sautė for a few minutes then set aside. Place your sausages and bacon into your air fryer and cook for 10-minutes. Place the baked beans into a ramekin and your (cracked) eggs in another ramekin and cook for an additional 10-minutes at 390°Fahrenheit. Serve warm.

Nutrition: calories 243, fat 12.3, carbs 10.5, protein 16.3

9. Morning Veggies on Toast

Preparation time: **5** minutes
Cooking time: **11** minutes
Servings: **4**

Ingredients:

1 tablespoon olive oil

½ cup soft goat cheese

2 tablespoons softened butter

4 slices French bread

2 green onions, sliced

1 small yellow squash, sliced

1 cup button mushrooms, sliced

1 red bell pepper, cut into strips

Directions:

Sprinkle your air fryer with olive oil and preheat it to 350°Fahrenheit. Mix the red bell peppers, squash, mushrooms and green onions, cook them for 7-minutes. Place vegetables on a plate and set aside. Spread the bread slices with butter and place into air fryer, with butter side up. Toast for 4-minutes. Spread the goat cheese on toasted bread and top with veggies. Serve warm.

Nutrition: calories 243, fat 10.3, carbs 8.5, protein 9.3

10. Rice Paper Bacon

Preparation time: **10** minutes
Cooking time: **30** minutes
Servings: **4**

 Ingredients:

4 pieces white rice paper,
cut into 1-inch thick strips

2 tablespoons water

2 tablespoons liquid smoke

2 tablespoons cashew butter

3 tablespoons soy sauce or tamari

 Directions:

Preheat your air fryer to 350°Fahrenheit. In a mixing bowl, add soy sauce, cashew butter, liquid smoke, and water, mix well. Soak the rice paper in this mixture for 5 minutes. Place the rice paper in air fryer and do not overlap pieces. Air fry for 15-minutes or until crispy. Serve with steamed vegetables!

Nutrition: calories 232, fat 7.4, carbs 6.2, protein 7.3

11. Italian Breakfast Frittata

Preparation time: **7** minutes
Cooking time: **10** minutes
Servings: **2**

Ingredients:

4 cherry tomatoes, sliced into halves

½ Italian sausage, sliced

½ teaspoon Italian seasoning

3 eggs

2-ounces parmesan cheese, shredded

1 tablespoon parsley, chopped

Salt and pepper to taste

Directions:

Preheat your air fryer to 360°Fahrenheit. Put the sausage and cherry tomatoes into baking dish and cook for 5-minutes. Crack eggs into small bowl, add parsley, Italian seasoning and mix well by whisking. Pour egg mixture over sausage and cherry tomatoes and place back into air fryer to cook for an additional 5-minutes. Serve warm.

Nutrition: calories 242, fat 11.2, carbs 9.3, protein 12.3

12. Air Fryer Broccoli & Tofu Scramble

Preparation   time: **10**   minutes
Cooking   time: **30**   minutes
Servings: **3**

Ingredients:

4 cups broccoli florets
1 block tofu, chopped finely
2 ½ cups red potatoes, chopped
2 tablespoons olive oil
2 tablespoons tamari
1 teaspoon turmeric powder
½ teaspoon garlic powder
½ teaspoon onion powder
½ cup onion, chopped

Directions:

Preheat your air fryer to 400°Fahrenheit. Mix the potatoes in a bowl with half of the olive oil. Place the potatoes into a baking dish that will fit into your air fryer and cook them for 15-minutes. Combine the remaining olive oil, tofu, tamari, turmeric, garlic powder and onion powder. Stir in the chopped onions. Add the broccoli florets. Pour this mixture on top of the air-fried potatoes and cook for an additional 15-minutes. Serve warm.

*Nutrition: **calories 232, fat 12.3, carbs 5.6, protein 14.5***

13. Air Fried Vegan Breakfast Bread

Preparation time: **5** minutes
Cooking time: **10** minutes
Servings: **2**

Ingredients:

1 vegan bread loaf, large

2 teaspoons chives

2 tablespoons nutritional yeast

2 tablespoons garlic puree

2 tablespoons olive oil

Salt and pepper to taste

Directions:

Preheat your air fryer to 375°Fahrenheit. Slice the bread loaf (not all the way through). In a bowl, combine the garlic puree, olive oil, and nutritional yeast. Add this mixture on top of the bread loaf. Sprinkle loaf with chives and season with salt and pepper. Place loaf inside of your air fryer and cook for 10-minutes.

*Nutrition: **calories 252, fat 9.6, carbs 5.7, protein 7.5***

14.   Breakfast Banana Cookies

Preparation   time: **10**   **minutes**
Cooking   time: **20**   **minutes**
Servings: **6**

Ingredients:

3 ripe bananas

1 teaspoon vanilla extract

1/3 cup olive oil

1 cup dates, pitted and chopped

2 cups rolled oats

 Directions:

Preheat your air fryer to 350°Fahrenheit. In a bowl, mash bananas and add the rest of the ingredients and mix well. Allow ingredients to rest in the fridge for 10-minutes. Cut some parchment paper to fit inside of your air fryer basket. Drop teaspoonful of mixture on parchment paper, making sure not to overlap the cookies. Cook the cookies for 20-minutes and serve with some almond milk.

 *Nutrition: **calories 224, fat 7.3, carbs 6.2, protein 6.5***

15. Spinach Balls

Preparation time: **10** minutes
Cooking time: **20** minutes
Servings: **4**

Ingredients:

1 carrot, peeled and grated

2 slices of bread, toasted and make into breadcrumbs

1 tablespoon corn flour

1 tablespoon nutritional yeast

½ teaspoon garlic, minced

1 egg, beaten

½ teaspoon garlic powder

½ onion, chopped

1 package fresh spinach, blanched and chopped

Directions:

Blend ingredients in a bowl, except the breadcrumbs. Make small balls with mixture and roll them over the bread crumbs. Place the spinach balls in your air fryer at 390°Fahrenheit for a cook time of 10-minutes. Serve warm.

*Nutrition: **calories 262, fat 11.2, carbs 7.4, protein 7.8***

16. Breakfast Sugar-Free Maple Cinnamon Buns

Preparation time: **10** minutes
Cooking time: **30** minutes
Servings: **9**

Ingredients:

¾ cup unsweetened almond milk
4 tablespoons sugar-free maple syrup
½ cup pecan nuts, toasted
3 teaspoons cinnamon powder
1 ½ cups almond flour, sifted
1 cup whole grain flour, sifted
1 tablespoon coconut oil, melted
3 tablespoons water
1 tablespoon ground flaxseed
1 ½ tablespoons active yeast
2 ripe bananas, sliced
4 dates, pitted
¼ cup icing sugar

Directions:

Heat the almond milk to lukewarm and add the syrup and yeast. Allow the yeast to activate for about 10-minutes. Mix flaxseed and water separately to make egg replacement. Allow flaxseed to soak for 2-minutes. Add coconut oil. Pour the flaxseed mixture into yeast mixture. In another bowl, add both types of flour, and 2 teaspoons cinnamon powder.

Pour into the yeast-flaxseed mixture and combine until dough is formed. Knead the dough on a floured surface for about 10-minutes. Place the kneaded dough into a greased bowl and cover it with a tea towel. Leave in a warm and dark area to rise for 1 hour. Make the filling by mixing the pecans, dates and banana slices and remaining teaspoon of cinnamon powder. Preheat your air fryer to 390°Fahrenheit. Roll the risen dough on a floured surface until it is thin. Spread the pecan mixture over the dough. Roll dough and cut it into nine slices. Place inside of dish that will fit into your air fryer and cook for 30-minutes. Once cook time is completed, sprinkle with icing sugar.

Nutrition: **calories 276, fat 11.3, carbs 9.2, protein 11.5**

17. Pea Protein Breakfast

Preparation time: **10** minutes
Cooking time: **15** minutes
Servings: **4**

Ingredients:

1 cup almond flour

1 teaspoon baking powder

3 eggs

1 cup mozzarella cheese, shredded

½ cup chicken or turkey strips

3 tablespoons pea protein

1 cup cream cheese

1 cup almond milk

Directions:

Preheat the air fryer to 390°Fahrenheit. Mix all the ingredients in mixing bowl and stir with wooden spoon. Fill muffin cups with mixture ¾ full and bake for 15-minutes and enjoy!

*Nutrition: **calories 256, fat 12.2, carbs 11.3, protein 17.2***

18. Breakfast Cherry & Almond Bars

Preparation   time: **8**   **minutes**
Cooking   time: **17**   **minutes**
Servings: **8**

Ingredients:

2 cups old-fashioned oats

½ cup quinoa, cooked

½ cup chia seeds

½ cup prunes, pureed

¼ teaspoon salt

2 teaspoons liquid Stevia

¾ cup almond butter

½ cup dried cherries, chopped

½ cup almonds, sliced

Directions:

Preheat your air fryer to 375°Fahrenheit. In a large mixing bowl, add quinoa, chia seeds, oats, cherries, almonds. In a saucepan over medium heat melt almond butter, liquid Stevia and coconut oil for 2-minutes and stir to combine. Add salt and prunes and mix well. Pour into baking dish that will fit inside of your air fryer and cook for 15-minutes. Allow to cool for an hour once cook time is completed, then slice the bars and serve.

*Nutrition: **calories 264, fat 12.5, carbs 12, protein 6.8***

19. Bacon & Cheddar Scrambled Eggs

Preparation time: **5** minutes
Cooking time: **10** minutes
Servings: **6**

Ingredients:

¼ teaspoon onion powder

4 eggs, beaten

3-ounces bacon, cooked, chopped

½ cup cheddar cheese, grated

3 tablespoons Greek yogurt

¼ teaspoon garlic powder

Salt and pepper to taste

Directions:

Preheat your air fryer to 330°Fahrenheit. Whisk eggs in a bowl, add salt and pepper to taste along with yogurt, garlic powder, onion powder, cheese, and bacon, stir. Add the egg mixture into oven-proof baking dish. Place into air fryer and cook for 10-minutes. Scramble eggs and serve warm.

Nutrition: calories 253, fat 12.2, carbs 11.6, protein 15.2

20.   Salmon & Carrot Mix Breakfast

Preparation time: **10** minutes
Cooking time: **30** minutes
Servings: **3**

Ingredients:

1 lb. salmon, chopped

2 cups feta, crumbled

4 bread slices

3 tablespoons pickled red onion

2 cucumbers, sliced

1 carrot, shredded

Directions:

Add salmon and feta to a bowl. Add carrot, red onion and cucumber and mix well. In an oven-safe tray make a layer of bread and then pour the salmon mix over it. Cook in your air fryer at 300°Fahrenheit for 15-minutes.

Nutrition: calories 226, fat 10.2, carbs 7.3, protein 14.6

21. French Toast Sticks

Preparation time: **10** minutes
Cooking time: **5** minutes
Servings: **2**

Ingredients:

Pinch of salt
½ tsp. nutmeg
1 tsp. cinnamon
2 eggs, beaten
2 sliced bread, cut into 4 strips each
2 tbsps. butter
Maple syrup for garnish

Directions:
Preheat your air fryer to 350 degrees F.
Add salt, nutmeg and cinnamon to egg.
Spread butter on bread strips.
Dip in the egg mixture.
Cook in the air fryer for two minutes.
Pause and then flip to cook the other side for two more minutes or until golden brown.
Drizzle with maple syrup before serving.
Nutrition: calories 196, fat 10, carbs 6.4, protein 5

Chapter 3: Appetizers Recipes

22. Green Cabbage with Mint

Preparation time: **10** minutes
Cooking time: **20** minutes
Servings: **2**

Ingredients:

1/2 green cabbage

1 package fresh mint

1 minced garlic clove

1 lemon

1 pinch salt

Directions:

Wash and cut the cabbage and mint roughly.

Sauté garlic and salt in a pan with 500ml of water and cook in an air fryer for 20 minutes. Serve and enjoy!

Nutrition: calories 24, fat 0, carbs 4, protein 1

23. Seasoned Chicken Skewers

Preparation time: **15** minutes
Cooking time: **20** minutes
Servings: **5**

Ingredients:

1 kg chicken breast

250 ml 0% fat yogurt

1 tsp. ground pepper powder

1 tsp. turmeric

1 tsp. cumin powder

1 tsp. coriander powder

1 tsp. grated ginger

1 garlic clove, mashed

Directions:

Dip 25 wooden skewers in a little water, so they don't burn while baking.

Remove fat from chicken breast and cut into pieces.

Prepare the sauce with the yogurt and the spices.

Put the chicken pieces on the skewers and, in a deep dish, make them completely soaked.

Leave several hours or a whole night in the fridge.

Then place the skewers on a grill or barbecue plate and cook in an air fryer for 8 to 10 minutes until the chicken is soft and golden. Serve and enjoy!

Nutrition: calories 100, fat 4, carbs 1, protein 26

24. Thyme Chicken

Preparation time: 15 minutes
Cooking time: 1 hour 5 minutes
Servings: 4

Ingredients:

1 whole chicken

1 pack fresh thyme

2 shallots

3 yogurts with 0% fat

1/2 lemon

1 packet parsley

Some mint leaves

1 garlic clove

Black pepper and salt, to taste

Directions:

Cut chicken into pieces and season.

Add a good amount of water to the bottom compartment of a steaming pan, add salt and wait till it boils.

Spread half of thyme on top of pan.

Arrange the chicken pieces on the thyme.

Top with the rest of the thyme and the peeled and chopped shallots.

Close the lid and cook in an air fryer for 30 to 35 minutes from the moment steam starts to escape.

In the meantime, put the yogurts in a bowl, add the half lemon juice, the chopped and dried mint leaves, the finely cut garlic clove.

Add black pepper along with salt, set aside in the refrigerator until serving, as an accompaniment to the chicken. Enjoy!

Nutrition: calories 225, fat 10, carbs 8, protein 24

25. Chicken with Yogurt

Preparation time: 10 minutes
Cooking time: 1 hour 30 minutes
Servings: 4

Ingredients:

1 whole chicken

120 g chopped onion

2 fat-free yogurts

1/2 tsp. ginger powder

1/2 tsp. paprika

2 tsp. lemon juice

2 tsp. curry

1/2 lemon zest

Black pepper and salt

Directions:

Cut chicken, remove skin and place the pieces in a nonstick air fryer.

Put the remaining ingredients over the chicken and cover.

Let it cook in an air fryer for about 1 hour and 30 minutes over low heat.

Season to taste and, if necessary, remove the lid at the end of cooking to reduce the sauce.

Serve very hot. Enjoy!

Nutrition: calories 285, fat 12, carbs 5, protein 26

26. Chicken with Ginger

Preparation time: 15 minutes
Cooking time: 1 hour 5 minutes
Servings: 4

Ingredients:

1 whole chicken

2 large onions

3 garlic cloves

Some cloves

5 g ginger

Black pepper and salt, to taste

Directions:

Cut chicken into pieces.

Sauté onions and garlic cloves, peeled and chopped in a lightly greased air fryer over low heat in the air fryer.

Add the chicken pieces to which the cloves will have been fixed. Cover with water.

Add the grated ginger, black pepper, along with salt.

Cook in an air fryer on medium heat until water evaporates. Serve and enjoy!

Nutrition: calories 285, fat 10, carbs 5, protein 2.5

27. Sautéed Chicken with Pepper

Preparation time: **10** minutes
Cooking time: **31** minutes
Servings: **4**

Ingredients:

4 chicken breasts

6 small red onions or shallots

3 to 6 fresh peppers

4 garlic cloves

1 piece fresh ginger

1 leaf lemon balm

150 ml water

Black pepper and salt

Directions:

Remove the skin from the chicken breasts and cut each into eight pieces vertically.

Chop the onion into thin strips for decoration of the dish. Wash and peel peppers, onions or shallots, garlic, ginger root, and lemon balm leaf.

Beat the peppers, half the ginger, and the lemon balm in a blender. Reserve.

Beat the onions, garlic, and other half of ginger until mashed.

In a lightly oiled nonstick frying pan, sauté the mashed pepper for 1 to 2 minutes.

Add the chicken pieces, mix so that they are well wrapped in the puree.

Add water and incorporate into onion puree. Season adequately using salt along with pepper.

Cook in an air fryer over high heat for 5 minutes with the air fryer uncapped.

Serve hot with onion slices for decoration. Enjoy!

Nutrition: calories 231, fat 5, carbs 6, protein 39

28. Turnip Curry Soup

Servings: 2

Total Time: 1 Hour 5 Minutes

Preparation time: 10 minutes

Cooking time: 1 hour 5 minutes

Servings: 2

Ingredients:

1 kg turnip

1 onion

4 garlic cloves

1 pinch curry powder

900 ml lean chicken broth

A few drops tabasco

1/2 lemon

200 g fat free yogurt

70 g thin slices nonfat ham

2 sprigs finely chopped parsley or chives

1 pinch nutmeg

Black pepper and salt

Directions:

Peel and remove the central and hardest part of the turnips.

Peel the onion and chop it roughly.

Peel the cloves of garlic and chop.

Sauté onion and garlic at medium temperature.

Cover and cook for 5 minutes, and then add the turnips.

Mix, cover, and cook for 10 minutes in the air fryer.

Add the curry, mix well, and add the broth.

Cook for about 30 minutes until it begins to boil.

Beat everything in a blender: the soup should be very thin. Heat the spice.

Add a few drops of tabasco and half lemon juice.

Heat in the air fryer and add 150g of yogurt.

Meanwhile, fry the ham in its own broth in a frying pan.

Drain, transfer it to a sheet of paper towels, and crumple it with your fingers.

Serve the soup with some yogurt, sprinkle bacon, parsley, and nutmeg.

Nutrition: calories 193, fat 9, fiber 5, carbs 8, protein 6

29. Eggplant Salad

Preparation time: **10** minutes
Cooking time: **25** minutes
Servings: **2**

Ingredients:

2 large eggplants

1 tsp. vinegar

1 garlic clove

4 spring onions

1 shallot

2 parsley stalks

Black pepper and salt

Directions:

Peel and cut the eggplants into large pieces.

Cook in the air fryer over high heat with boiling water for about 20 minutes.

Lower the heat and cook for another 20 minutes.

Let cool and crush with a fork.

Drizzle the eggplant with a well-seasoned vinaigrette dressing with chopped garlic, chives, and shallot in very small pieces.

Sprinkle the chopped parsley and serve very cold.

Nutrition: calories 133, fat 12, carbs 5, protein 1.3

30. Greek-Style Lemon Soup

Preparation time: **5** minutes
Cooking time: **20** minutes
Servings: **2**

Ingredients:

1 L water

2 cubes fat-free chicken broth

1 pinch saffron

2 carrots

2 zucchinis

2 egg yolks

1 lemon

Directions:

Boil water with the chicken broth cubes and saffron.

Meanwhile, grate the carrot and zucchini roughly.

Add the carrot to the broth and simmer for 5 minutes.

Add zucchini and boil for 3 minutes.

Add one or two egg yolks, zest, and lemon juice.

Keep on medium heat in the air fryer so as not to boil anymore.

Nutrition: calories 70, fat 0, carbs 10, protein 6

31. Zucchini Tajine

Preparation time: **20** minutes
Cooking time: **40** minutes
Servings: **2**

Ingredients:

2 garlic cloves

1 tsp. cumin powder

1 tsp. coriander powder

1 tsp. garam masala powder

500 ml water

1 cube chicken broth without fat

2 tbsp. tomato paste

4 zucchinis

For Garnishing:

1 lemon

1 bunch coriander

Directions:

Sauté minced garlic and spices in a large saucepan in the air fryer over low heat for a few minutes.

Add the water, the chicken stock cube, the tomato extract, and the sliced zucchini.

Cook for 35 minutes at medium temperature topped with pan and serve it with lemon and cilantro sauce, if possible, in a tajine pan.

Nutrition: calories 207, fat 16, carbs 6, protein 9

32. Eggplant Terrine

Preparation time: 20 minutes
Cooking time: 1 hour 30 minutes
Servings: 4

Ingredients:

2 eggplants

100 g chicken or turkey ham

3 sprigs celery1 garlic clove

3 sprigs chopped parsley

3 tomatoes

Directions:

Slice the eggplants and sprinkle salt to remove excess water.

Sauté diced ham in the air fryer.

Reserve. Save the cooking stock for the vegetables.

Cut the celery branches and sauté them in the pan over low heat.

Mix ham and celery.

In an air fryer proof dish, make a layer of sliced eggplant, one with a mixture of chopped ham, celery, parsley, and garlic, one with sliced tomatoes, and one with the remaining eggplant slices.

Cook for 1 hour at 180 degrees.

Nutrition: calories 262, fat 27, carbs 6, protein 15

33. Garden Terrine

Preparation time: **5** minutes
Cooking time: **25** minutes
Servings: **4**

Ingredients:

900 g carrots
500 g leeks
5 beaten eggs
125 g 0% fat cottage chees
100 g chopped nonfat ham
Black pepper and salt

Directions:

Steam the leek beforehand.

Grate the carrot and beat previously cooked leek in a blender.

Mix in beaten eggs, cottage cheese, black pepper, along with salt.

Add the vegetables, mix well, and put them in a rectangular pan.

Cook in the air fryer without lid in the preheated air fryer to 190 degrees, and follow the cooking regularly.

Nutrition: calories 300, fat 12, carbs 6, protein 15

34. Parsley Tomatoes

Preparation time: **10** minutes
Cooking time: **18** minutes
Servings: **2**

Ingredients:

4 ripe tomatoes
1 red or white onion, cut into 8 equal parts
2 minced garlic cloves
5 jalapeno peppers
1 1/2 L lemon juice
Some coriander stalks
A pinch salt

Directions:

Cook tomatoes in the air fryer for 30 seconds.

Peel and remove the seeds in the mixer container.

Put the onion pieces, the garlic, and the salt.

Remove the peduncle from the jalapeno peppers and cut them in two.

Save some seeds for a more or less spicy sauce.

Cut the peppers roughly and add the desired amount of seeds to the mixer bowl.

Grind until the sauce reaches the desired consistency.

Transfer the sauce to a pan and cook in the air fryer at medium temperature until it is covered in a pink foam, which should take about 6 to 8 minutes to cook.

Remove from heat and let cool for at least 10 minutes.

Add lemon juice and coriander.

Nutrition: calories 57, fat 0, carbs 6, protein 3

35. Eggplants with Garlic and Parsley

Preparation time: **15** minutes
Cooking time: **30** minutes
Servings: **2**

Ingredients:

200 to 250 g eggplant

1 garlic clove

2 parsley stalks

Black pepper and salt, to taste

Direction

Remove the stalks, wash, and dry the eggplants.

Cut them in two lengthwise. Remove the pulp from the eggplants.

Chop the garlic, parsley and eggplant pulp.

Season adequately using salt along with pepper.

Fill the eggplants with the mixture.

Close them in foil and cook in the air fryer for about 30 to 35 minutes at 170 degrees.

Nutrition: calories 110, fat 10, carbs 3, protein 1

36. Air Fryer Eggplants

Preparation time: **10** minutes
Cooking time: **35** minutes
Servings: **1**

Ingredients:

1 eggplant

1 tomato

1 medium onion

1 garlic clove

2 thyme stems

1 tbsp. basil

Black pepper and salt, to taste

Directions:

Wash and dice the eggplant. Wash and mash the tomato.

Peel the onion and chop the garlic.

Sauté onion with some water until translucent.

Add the eggplant and brown in the air fryer over high heat and then medium.

Add the tomatoes, garlic, thyme, and basil.

Season adequately using salt along with pepper.

Cover and cook in the air fryer for 30 minutes over low heat.

Nutrition: calories 110, fat 10, carbs 3, protein 1

37. Vegetable Broth

Preparation time: **6** minutes
Cooking time: **15** minutes
Servings: **1**

Ingredients:

50 g carrots

50 g mushrooms

25 g celery sprigs

25 g leeks, white

2 medium tomatoes

1 1/4 L fat free chicken broth

1 packet parsley

Salt and pepper, to taste

Directions:

Cut the washed and peeled vegetables into very thin sticks. Cut the tomatoes in four.

Remove seeds and water, then roughly cut into cubes.

Wait till it boils in the air fryer, sprinkle black pepper and salt as per your taste.

Dip the vegetables (minus the tomatoes) in the stock and cook them in the air fryer without covering the pan for 5 to 6 minutes (the vegetables should be slightly crispy).

Remove the pan from the heat, add the tomato pieces and the finely chopped parsley.

Serve it hot.

Nutrition: calories 70, fat 5, carbs 4, protein 2

38. Greek-Style Mushrooms

Preparation time: **10** minutes
Cooking time: **20** minutes
Servings: **2**

Ingredients:

5 tsp. lemon juice

2 bay leaves

1 tsp. coriander seeds

1 tsp. black pepper

700 g mushrooms

4 tsp. minced parsley

Salt, to taste

Directions:

Add a liter of water in a saucepan with lemon juice, bay leaves, coriander seeds, and black pepper. Season with salt.

Wait till it boils and cook in the air fryer for 10 minutes.

Remove the grounded part of the champignon's feet. Wash quickly, drain and cut into pieces.

Add the mushrooms to the pan and wait for it to boil again.

Set 2 minutes and turn off the heat.

Add the parsley. Mix gently. Let it cool completely in the broth.

Drain the mushrooms, put them on a plate, and drizzle with the cooking broth, adding some coriander grains.

Nutrition: calories 60, fat 8, carbs 2, protein 5

39. Zucchini Fondue with Lobsters

Preparation time: 10 minutes
Cooking time: 1 hour 5 minutes
Servings: 4

Ingredients:

1 kg cooked lobster

800 g zucchini

2 large onions

6 sprigs mint

1 tbsp. olive oil

1/2 lemon juice

Salt and pepper, to taste

Gray coarse sea salt, or common coarse salt

Directions:

Wash the zucchini, dry, peel, and cut into 5mm strips.

Peel and chop the onions. Heat the olive oil in a pan and Sauté the onion.

Add the zucchini, salt along with pepper, mix and cook in the air fryer for 40 minutes, stir the total time required to prepare occasionally so as not to stick to the bottom, and when the mixture becomes tender, add the lemon juice and minced mint.

Arrange zucchini fondue and lobster meat on a serving platter.

Nutrition: calories 250, fat 17, carbs 5, protein 15

40. Cooked Tuna

Preparation time: **5** minutes
Cooking time: **20** minutes
Servings: **4**

Ingredients:

2 parsley leaves
1 small packet fresh oregano
1 small packet thyme
3 to 4 bay leaves
1 lemon
1 tsp. mustard seed
1 tuna slice, about 400 to 500 g

Directions:

In a container, finely chop herbs and mash bay leaves.
Add lemon juice and mustard grains. Mix well.
Pass both sides of the tuna slice in the marinade.
Cook the fish in the air fryer for 5 minutes (or in a lightly oiled frying pan) on each side over high heat and drizzle with the marinade.

Nutrition: calories 128, fat 3, carbs 0, protein 24

41. Crab Crepes

Preparation time: **5** minutes
Cooking time: **10** minutes
Servings: **2**

Ingredients:

3 eggs

170 g shredded crab meat

2 tbsp. mustard

Directions:

Mix ingredients, make balls and crush with the palm of your hand to flatten into a disc.

Cook in an air fryer for 10 minutes. Serve

Nutrition: calories 225, fat 10, carbs 3, protein 18

Chapter 4. Seafood Recipes

42. Salmon and Orange Marmalade

Preparation time: **10 minutes**
Cooking time: 15 minutes
Servings: 4
Ingredients:
1 pound wild salmon, skinless, boneless and cubed
2 lemons, sliced
¼ cup balsamic vinegar
¼ cup orange juice
1/3 cup orange marmalade
A pinch of salt and black pepper
Directions:
Heat up a pot with the vinegar over medium heat, add marmalade and orange juice, stir, bring to a simmer, cook for 1 minute and take off heat.

Thread salmon cubes and lemon slices on skewers, season with salt and black pepper, brush them with half of the orange marmalade mix, arrange in your air fryer's basket and cook at 360 degrees F for 3 minutes on each side.

Brush skewers with the rest of the vinegar mix, divide among plates and serve right away with a side salad.
Enjoy!
Nutrion: calories 240, fat 9, carbs 14, protein 10

43. Chili Salmon

Preparation time: **10 minutes**

Cooking time: 15 minutes

Servings: 12

Ingredients:

1 and ¼ cups coconut, shredded

1 pound salmon, cubed

1/3 cup flour

A pinch of salt and black pepper

1 egg

2 tablespoons olive oil

¼ cup water

4 red chilies, chopped

3 garlic cloves, minced

¼ cup balsamic vinegar

½ cup honey

Directions:

In a bowl, mix flour with a pinch of salt and stir.

In another bowl, mix egg with black pepper and whisk.

Put coconut in a third bowl.

Dip salmon cubes in flour, egg and coconut, put them in your air fryer's basket, cook at 370 degrees F for 8 minutes, shaking halfway and divide among plates.

Heat up a pan with the water over medium high heat, add chilies, cloves, vinegar and honey, stir very well, bring to a boil, simmer for a couple of minutes, drizzle over salmon and serve.

Nutrition: calories 220, fat 12, carbs 14, protein 13

44. Salmon and Lemon Relish

Preparation time: **10 minutes**

Cooking time: 30 minutes

Servings: 2

Ingredients:

fillets

Salt and black pepper

1 tablespoon oil

lemon juice

shallot

lemon

parsley

oil

Directions:

Season salmon with salt and pepper, rub with 1 tablespoon oil, place in your air fryer's basket and cook at 320 degrees F for 20 minutes, flipping the fish halfway.

Meanwhile, in a bowl, mix shallot with the lemon juice, a pinch of salt and black pepper, stir and leave aside for 10 minutes.

In a separate bowl, mix marinated shallot with lemon slices, salt, pepper, parsley and ¼ cup oil and whisk well.

Divide salmon on plates, top with lemon relish and serve.

Nutrition: calories 200, fat 3, carbs 23, protein 19

45. Salmon and Avocado Sauce

Preparation time: **10 minutes**

Cooking time: 10 minutes

Servings: 4

Ingredients:

1 avocado, pitted, peeled and chopped

4 salmon fillets, boneless

¼ cup cilantro, chopped

1/3 cup coconut milk

1 tablespoon lime juice

1 tablespoon lime zest, grated

1 teaspoon onion powder

1 teaspoon garlic powder

Salt and black pepper to the taste

Directions:

Season salmon fillets with salt, black pepper and lime zest, rub well, put in your air fryer, cook at 350 degrees F for 9 minutes, flipping once and divide among plates.

In your food processor, mix avocado with cilantro, garlic powder, onion powder, lime juice, salt, pepper and coconut milk, blend well, drizzle over salmon and serve right away.

Nutrition: calories 260, fat 7, carbs 28, protein 18

46. Crusted Salmon

Preparation time: **10 minutes**

Cooking time: **10 minutes**

Servings: 4

Ingredients:

1 cup pistachios, chopped

4 salmon fillets

¼ cup lemon juice

2 tablespoons honey

1 teaspoon dill, chopped

Salt and black pepper to the taste

1 tablespoon mustard

Directions:

In a bowl, mix pistachios with mustard, honey, lemon juice, salt, black pepper and dill, whisk and spread over salmon.

Put in your air fryer and cook at 350 degrees F for 10 minutes.

Divide among plates and serve with a side salad.

Nutrition: calories 300, fat 17, fiber 12, carbs 20, protein 22

47. Stuffed Calamari

Preparation time: **10 minutes**

Cooking time: 25 minutes

Servings: 4

Ingredients:

4 big calamari, tentacles separated and chopped and tubes reserved

2 tablespoons parsley, chopped

5 ounces kale, chopped

2 garlic cloves, minced

1 red bell pepper, chopped

1 tablespoon olive oil

2 ounces canned tomato puree

1 yellow onion, chopped

Salt and black pepper to the taste

Directions:

Heat up a pan with the oil over medium heat, add onion and garlic, stir and cook for 2 minutes.

Add bell pepper, tomato puree, calamari tentacles, kale, salt and pepper, stir, cook for 10 minutes and take off heat. stir and cook for 3 minutes.

Stuff calamari tubes with this mix, secure with toothpicks, put in your air fryer and cook at 360 degrees F for 20 minutes.

Divide calamari on plates, sprinkle parsley all over and serve.

Nutrition: calories 322, fat 10, carbs 14, protein 22

48. Tuna Kabobs

Preparation time: **5 minutes**

Cooking time: 12 minutes

Servings: 4

Ingredients:

1 pound tuna steaks, boneless and cubed

1 chili pepper, minced

4 green onions, chopped

2 tablespoons lime juice

A drizzle of olive oil

Salt and black pepper to the taste

Directions:

In a bowl mix all the ingredients.

Thread the tuna cubes on skewers, arrange them in your air fryer's basket and cook at 370 degrees F for 12 minutes.

Divide between plates and serve with a side salad.

Nutrition: calories 226, fat 12, carbs 4, protein 15

49. Cod and Tomatoes

Preparation time: **5 minutes**

Cooking time: 15 minutes

Servings: 4

Ingredients:

1 cup cherry tomatoes, halved

Salt and black pepper to the taste

2 tablespoons olive oil

4 cod fillets, skinless and boneless

2 tablespoons cilantro, chopped

Directions:

In a baking dish that fits your air fryer, mix all the ingredients, introduce in your air fryer and cook at 370 degrees F for 15 minutes.

Divide everything between plates and serve right away.

Nutrition: calories 248, fat 11, carbs 5, protein 11

50. Tilapia and Tomato Mix

Preparation time: **5 minutes**
Cooking time: 20 minutes
Servings: 4
Ingredients:
4 tilapia fillets, boneless and halved
Salt and black pepper to the taste
1 cup roasted peppers, chopped
¼ cup tomato paste
1 cup tomatoes, cubed
1 tablespoon lemon juice
2 tablespoons olive oil
1 teaspoon garlic powder
1 teaspoon oregano, dried
Directions:
In a baking dish that fits your air fryer, mix the fish with all the other ingredients, heave, introduce in your air fryer and cook at 380 degrees F for 20 minutes.
Divide into bowls and serve.
Nutrition: calories 250, fat 9, carbs 5, protein 14

51. Shrimp and Lemon Vinaigrette

Preparation time: **5 minutes**

Cooking time: 12 minutes

Servings: 4

Ingredients:

1 and ½ pounds shrimp, peeled and deveined

Zest of ½ lemon, grated

Juice of ½ lemon

A pinch of salt and black pepper

2 tablespoons mustard

2 tablespoons olive oil

2 tablespoons parsley, chopped

Directions:

In a bowl, mix all the ingredients and toss well.

Put the shrimp in your air fryer's basket and reserve the lemon vinaigrette.

Cook at 350 degrees F for 12 minutes, flipping the shrimp halfway, divide between plates and serve with reserved vinaigrette drizzled on top.

Nutrition: calories 202, fat 8, carbs 5, protein 14

52. Garlic Shrimp

Preparation time: **5 minutes**
Cooking time: 12 minutes
Servings: 4
Ingredients:
1 pound shrimp, peeled and deveined
1 teaspoon cumin, ground
2 tablespoons parsley, chopped
2 tablespoons olive oil
A pinch of salt and black pepper
4 garlic cloves, minced
1 tablespoon lime juice
Directions:
In a pan that fits your air fryer, mix all the ingredients, put the pan in your air fryer and cook at 370 degrees F and cook for 12 minutes, shaking the fryer halfway.
Divide into bowls and serve.
Nutrition: calories 220, fat 11, carbs 5, protein 12

53. Shrimp and Green Beans

Preparation time: **5 minutes**

Cooking time: 15 minutes

Servings: **4**

Ingredients:

1 pound shrimp, peeled and deveined

A pinch of salt and black pepper

½ pound green beans, trimmed and halved

Juice of 1 lime

2 tablespoons cilantro, chopped

¼ cup ghee, melted

Directions:

In a pan that fits your air fryer, mix all the ingredients, introduce in the fryer and cook at 360 degrees F for 15 minutes shaking the fryer halfway.

Divide into bowls and serve.

Nutrition: calories 222, fat 8, carbs 5, protein 10

54. Sesame Shrimp

Preparation time: **3 minutes**

Cooking time: 12 minutes

Servings: 4

Ingredients:

1 pound shrimp

A pinch of salt and black pepper

1 tablespoon sesame seeds, toasted

½ teaspoon Italian seasoning

olive oil

Directions:

In a bowl, mix the shrimp with the rest of the ingredients and toss well.

Put the shrimp in the air fryer's basket, cook at 370 degrees F for 12 minutes, divide into bowls and serve,

Nutrition: calories 199, fat 11, fiber 2, carbs 4, protein 11

55. Hot Basil Cod

Preparation time: **5 minutes**

Cooking time: 15 minutes

Servings: 4

Ingredients:

4 cod fillets, boneless

1 teaspoon red pepper flakes

½ teaspoon hot paprika

2 tablespoon olive oil

1 teaspoon basil, dried

Salt and black pepper to the taste

Directions:

In a bowl, mix the cod with all the other ingredients and toss.

Put the fish in your air fryer's basket and cook at 380 degrees F for 15 minutes.

Divide the cod between plates and serve.

Nutrition: calories 194, fat 7, fiber 2, carbs 4, protein 12

56. Rosemary Shrimp and Tomatoes

Preparation time: **5 minutes**

Cooking time: 12 minutes

Servings: 4

Ingredients:

1 pound shrimp, peeled and deveined

1 cup cherry tomatoes, halved

4 garlic cloves, minced

Salt and black pepper to the taste

1 tablespoon rosemary, chopped

2 tablespoons ghee, melted

Directions:

In a pan that fits the air fryer, mix all the ingredients, put the pan in the fryer and cook at 380 degrees F for 12 minutes.

Divide into bowls and serve hot.

Nutrition: calories 220, fat 14, fiber 2, carbs 6, protein 15

57. Shrimp and Pesto

Preparation time: **5 minutes**

Cooking time: 12 minutes

Servings: 4

Ingredients:

½ cup parsley leaves

½ cup basil leaves

2 tablespoons lemon juice

1/3 cup pine nuts

¼ cup parmesan, grated

A pinch of salt and black pepper

½ cup olive oil

1 and ½ pounds shrimp, peeled and deveined

¼ teaspoon lemon zest, grated

Directions:

In a blender, combine all the ingredients except the shrimp and pulse well.

In a bowl, mix the shrimp with the pesto and toss.

Put the shrimp in your air fryer's basket and cook at 360 degrees F for 12 minutes, flipping the shrimp halfway.

Divide the shrimp into bowls and serve.

Nutrition: calories 240, fat 10, carbs 4, protein 12

58. Salmon and Green Olives

Preparation time: **5 minutes**

Cooking time: 15 minutes

Servings: 4

Ingredients:

1 tablespoon lemon zest, grated

1/3 cup olive oil

4 salmon fillets, boneless

1 cup green olives, pitted and sliced

Juice of 2 limes

Salt and black pepper to the taste

Directions:

In a baking dish that fits your air fryer, mix all the ingredients, put the pan in the fryer and cook at 370 degrees F for 15 minutes.

Divide everything between plates and serve.

Nutrition: calories 204, fat 12, carbs 5, protein 15

59. Shrimp and Zucchinis

Preparation time: **5 minutes**

Cooking time: 15 minutes

Servings: 4

Ingredients:

1 pound shrimp

A pinch of salt and black pepper

2 zucchinis, cut into medium cubes

1 tablespoon lemon juice

olive oil

1 tablespoon garlic, minced

Directions:

In a pan that fits the air fryer, combine all the ingredients, put the pan in the machine and cook at 370 degrees F for 15 minutes.

Divide between plates and serve right away.

Nutrition: calories 221, fat 9, carbs 15, protein 11

60. Shrimp and Black Olives

Preparation time: **5 minutes**

Cooking time: 12 minutes

Servings: 4

Ingredients:

1 pound shrimp

4 garlic clove, minced

1 cup black olives, pitted and chopped

3 tablespoons parsley

olive oil

Directions:

In a pan that fits the air fryer, combine all the ingredients, put the pan in the machine and cook at 370 degrees F for 12 minutes.

Divide between plates and serve.

Nutrition: calories 251, fat 12, carbs 6, protein 15

61. Salmon And Cauliflower Rice

Preparation time: **5 minutes**

Cooking time: **25 minutes**

Servings: 4

Ingredients:

4 salmon fillets, boneless

Salt and black pepper to the taste

1 cup cauliflower, riced

½ cup chicken stock

1 teaspoon turmeric powder

1 tablespoon butter, melted

Directions:

In a pan that fits your air fryer, mix the cauliflower rice with the other ingredients except the salmon and toss.

Arrange the salmon fillets over the cauliflower rice, put the pan in the fryer and cook at 360 degrees F for 25 minutes, flipping the fish after 15 minutes.

Divide everything between plates and serve.

Nutrition: calories 241, fat 12, carbs 6, protein 12

62. **Trout** and Mint Mix

Preparation time: **5 minutes**

Cooking time: **16 minutes**

Servings: 4

Ingredients:

4 rainbow trout

1 cup olive oil+ 3 tablespoons

Juice of 1 lemon

A pinch of salt and black pepper

1 cup parsley, chopped

3 garlic cloves, minced

½ cup mint, chopped

Zest of 1 lemon

1/3 pine nuts

1 avocado, peeled, pitted and roughly chopped

Directions:

Pat dry the trout, season with salt and pepper and rub with 3 tablespoons oil.

Put the fish in your air fryer's basket and cook for 8 minutes on each side.

Divide the fish between plates and drizzle half of the lemon juice all over.

In a blender, combine the rest of the oil with the remaining lemon juice, parsley, garlic, mint, lemon zest, pine nuts and the avocado and pulse well.

Spread this over the trout and serve.

Nutrition: calories 240, fat 12, carbs 6, protein 9

63. **Seafood** Stew

Preparation Time: **10 minutes**
Cooking Time: 30 Minutes
Servings: 4
Ingredients:
5 oz. white rice
3 oz. sea bass fillet; skinless, boneless and chopped.
2 oz. peas
1 red bell pepper; chopped.
14 oz. white wine
3 oz. water
2 oz. squid pieces
7 oz. mussels
6 scallops
4 shrimp
4 crayfish
1 tbsp. olive oil
Salt and black pepper to the taste
Directions:
In your air fryer's pan; mix sea bass with shrimp, mussels, scallops, crayfish, clams and squid.
Add the oil, salt and pepper and toss to coat.
In a bowl; mix peas salt, pepper, bell pepper and rice and stir.
Add this over seafood, also add wine and water, place pan in your air fryer and cook at 400 °F, for 20 minutes; stirring halfway. Divide into bowls and serve for lunch.
Nutrition: Calories: 300, Fat: 12, Carbs: 23, Protein: 25

Chapter 5. Poultry Recipes

64. Mozzarella Chicken Breasts

Preparation time: **5 minutes**

Cooking time: 24 minutes

Servings: 6

Ingredients:

6 chicken breasts, skinless, boneless and halved

A pinch of salt and black pepper

2 tablespoons olive oil

1 pound mozzarella, sliced

2 cups baby spinach

1 teaspoon Italian seasoning

2 tomatoes, sliced

1 tablespoon basil, chopped

Directions:

Make slits in each chicken breast halves, season with salt, pepper and Italian seasoning and stuff with mozzarella, spinach and tomatoes.

Drizzle the oil over stuffed chicken, put it in your air fryer's basket and cook at 370 degrees F for 12 minutes on each side.

Divide between plates and serve with basil sprinkled on top.

Nutrition: calories 285, fat 12, carbs 7, protein 15

65. Smoked Chicken Wings

Preparation time: **5 minutes**

Cooking time: **30 minutes**

Servings: **4**

Ingredients:

1 tablespoon olive oil

2 pounds chicken wings

1 tablespoon lime juice

2 teaspoons smoked paprika

1 teaspoon red pepper flakes, crushed

Salt and black pepper to the taste

Directions:

In a bowl, mix the chicken wings with all the other ingredients and toss well.

Put the chicken wings in your air fryer's basket and cook at 380 degrees F for 15 minutes on each side.

Divide between plates and serve with a side salad.

Nutrition: calories 280, fat 13, carbs 6, protein 14

66. Crispy Chicken Tenders

Preparation time: **5 minutes**

Cooking time: 20 minutes

Servings: 4

Ingredients:

4 chicken breasts, skinless, boneless and cut into tenders

A pinch of salt and black pepper

1/3 cup almond flour

2 eggs, whisked

9 ounces coconut flakes

Directions:

Season the chicken tenders with salt and pepper, dredge them in almond flour, then dip in eggs and roll in coconut flakes.

Put the chicken tenders in your air fryer's basket and cook at 400 degrees F for 10 minutes on each side.

Divide between plates and serve with a side salad.

Nutrition: calories 250, fat 12, carbs 6, protein 15

67. Marinated Drumsticks

Preparation time: **10 minutes**

Cooking time: 30 minutes

Servings: 4

Ingredients:

1 and ½ cups tomato sauce

1 teaspoon onion powder

A pinch of salt and black pepper

1 tablespoon coconut aminos

½ teaspoon chili powder

2 pounds chicken drumsticks

Directions:

In bowl, mix the chicken drumsticks with all the other ingredients, and keep in the fridge for 10 minutes.

Drain the drumsticks, put them in your air fryer's basket and cook at 370 degrees F for 15 minutes on each side.

Divide everything between plates and serve.

Nutrition: calories 254, fat 14, carbs 6, protein 15

68. Nutmeg Chicken Thighs

Preparation time: **5 minutes**

Cooking time: 30 minutes

Servings: 4

Ingredients:

2 pounds chicken thighs

A pinch of salt and black pepper

2 tablespoons olive oil

½ teaspoon nutmeg, ground

Directions:

Season the chicken thighs with salt and pepper, and rub with the rest of the ingredients.

Put the chicken thighs in air fryer's basket, cook at 360 degrees F for 15 minutes on each side, divide between plates and serve.

Nutrition: calories 271, fat 12, carbs 6, protein 13

69. Chives Chicken Tenders

Preparation time: **5 minutes**

Cooking time: 20 minutes

Servings: 4

Ingredients:

1 pound chicken tenders, boneless, skinless

A pinch of salt and black pepper

Juice of 1 lemon

1 tablespoon chives, chopped

A drizzle of olive oil

Directions:

In a bowl, mix the chicken tenders with all ingredients except the chives, toss, put the meat in your air fryer's basket and cook at 370 degrees F for 10 minutes on each side.

Divide between plates and serve with chives sprinkled on top.

Nutrition: calories 230, fat 13, carbs 6, protein 16

70. Turmeric Chicken Wings Mix

Preparation time: **5 minutes**

Cooking time: 30 minutes

Servings: 4

Ingredients:

2 pounds chicken wings, halved

¼ cup red vinegar

4 garlic cloves, minced

Salt and black pepper to the taste

4 tablespoons olive oil

1 tablespoon garlic powder

1 teaspoon turmeric powder

Directions:

In a bowl, mix the chicken with all the other ingredients and toss well.

Put the chicken wings in your air fryer's basket and cook at 370 degrees F for 30 minutes, flipping the meat halfway.

Divide everything between plates and serve with a side salad.

Nutrition: calories 250, fat 12, carbs 6, protein 15

71. Turkey Breasts and Fresh Herbs Mix

Preparation time: **10 minutes**

Cooking time: 25 minutes

Servings: 4

Ingredients:

2 turkey breasts, skinless, boneless and halved

4 tablespoons butter, melted

2 tablespoons thyme, chopped

2 tablespoons sage, chopped

1 tablespoons rosemary, chopped

2 tablespoons parsley, chopped

A pinch of salt and black pepper

2 cups chicken stock

2 celery stalks, chopped

Directions:

Heat up a pan that fits your air fryer with the butter over medium-high heat, add the turkey and brown for 2-3 minutes on each side.

Add the herbs, stock, celery, salt and pepper, toss, put the pan in your air fryer, cook at 390 degrees F for 20 minutes.

Divide between plates and serve.

Nutrition: calories 284, fat 14, carbs 6, protein 20

72. Turkey and Rosemary Butter

Preparation time: **5 minutes**

Cooking time: **24 minutes**

Servings: 4

Ingredients:

1 turkey breast

A pinch of salt and black pepper

Juice of 1 lemon

2 tablespoons rosemary, chopped

2 tablespoons butter, melted

Directions:

In a bowl, mix the butter with the rosemary, lemon juice, salt and pepper and whisk really well.

Brush the turkey pieces with the rosemary butter, put them your air fryer's basket, cook at 380 degrees F for 12 minutes on each side.

Divide between plates and serve with a side salad.

Nutrition: calories 236, fat 12, carbs 6, protein 13

73. Turkey and Shallot Sauce

Preparation time: **5 minutes**
Cooking time: 30 minutes
Servings: 4
Ingredients:
1 big turkey breast
1 tablespoon olive oil
¼ teaspoon sweet paprika
Salt and black pepper to the taste
1 cup chicken stock
3 tablespoons butter, melted
4 shallots, chopped
Directions:
Heat up a pan that fits the air fryer with the olive oil and the butter over medium high heat, add the turkey cubes, and brown for 3 minutes on each side.
Add the shallots, stir and sauté for 5 minutes more.
Add the paprika, stock, salt and pepper, toss, put the pan in the air fryer and cook at 370 degrees F for 20 minutes.
Divide into bowls and serve.
Nutrition: calories 236, fat 12, fiber 4, carbs 6, protein 15

74. Mustard Turkey Bites

Preparation time: **5 minutes**
Cooking time: 20 minutes
Servings: 4
Ingredients:
1 big turkey breast
4 garlic cloves, minced
Salt and black pepper to the taste
1 and ½ tablespoon olive oil
1 tablespoon mustard
Directions:
In a bowl, mix the chicken with the garlic and the other ingredients and toss.

Put the turkey in your air fryer's basket, cook at 360 degrees F for 20 minutes, divide between plates and serve with a side salad.

Nutrition: calories 240, fat 12, carbs 6, protein 15

75. Balsamic Glazed Turkey

Preparation time: **5 minutes**

Cooking time: 30 minutes

Servings: 4

Ingredients:

1 big turkey breast

3 tablespoons balsamic vinegar

2 garlic cloves, minced

3 tablespoons butter, melted

A pinch of salt and black pepper

1 tablespoon chives, chopped

Directions:

Heat up a pan that fits the air fryer with the butter over medium-high heat, add the garlic and sauté for 2 minutes.

Add the turkey, brown for 2 minutes on each side and take off the heat.

Add the rest of the ingredients, toss, put the pan in your air fryer and cook at 380 degrees F for 20 minutes.

Divide everything between plates and serve.

Nutrition: calories 283, fat 12, carbs 5, protein 15

Conclusion

Thanks for reading through this book. It is my desire that by now the purpose of this recipe book has been realized that was to show you the versatility of the air fryer. When it comes to cooking and using a new kitchen appliance is learning the ins and out; the way that it cooks foods specifically. If you've read through this book and tried your hand at a variety of the recipes, then you should by now know what using the air fryer entails.

The next step is to start putting that air fryer to good use. You have spent some good money on the air fryer in the hopes that it can make your life at least a little bit easier, so now it is time to find the good recipes that will make this a reality. There are a lot of good recipes to choose; the trick is to just find the ones that will hit the spot with your family and will have even those picky eaters coming back for seconds and even thirds. This guidebook will provide you with this benefit in no time.

Inside this guidebook, we will take a look at some of the steps that you can follow in order to get started using your air fryer. Are you looking for a tasty breakfast that will bring the family together before they run out the door to the next adventure? Are you interested in finding something for a snack on the go, a good lunch that doesn't include fast food, or even dinner for those busy nights or the ones that you want to slow down with and enjoy the company of your family? You will find these recipes and more inside!

This is just the start. There really are no limits to working with the air fryer, and we will explore some more recipes as well. In addition to all the great options that we talked about before, you will find that there are tasty desserts that can help that sweet tooth in no time, and some great sauces and dressing so you can always be in control over the foods you eat. There are just so many options to choose from that it won't take long before you find a whole bunch of recipes to use, and before you start to wonder why you didn't get the air fryer so much sooner.

www.ingramcontent.com/pod-product-compliance
Lightning Source LLC
Chambersburg PA
CBHW062135020426
42335CB00013B/1224

9781990334016